Plague and Other Yersinia Infections

CURRENT TOPICS IN INFECTIOUS DISEASE

Series Editors:

William B. Greenough III
Division of Geographic Medicine
The Johns Hopkins University School of Medicine
Baltimore, Maryland

Thomas C. Merigan
Head, Division of Infectious Disease
Stanford University Medical Center
Stanford, California

The Atypical Mycobacteria and Human Mycobacteriosis
John S. Chapman

Infections of the Gastrointestinal Tract: Microbiology, Pathophysiology, and Clinical Features
Herbert L. DuPont and Larry K. Pickering

Coccidioidomycosis: A Text
Edited by David A. Stevens

Cytomegalovirus: Biology and Infection
Monto Ho

Infective Endocarditis and Other Intravascular Infections
Lawrence R. Freedman

Plague and Other Yersinia Infections
Thomas Butler

A Continuation Order Plan is available for this series. A continuation order will bring delivery of each new volume immediately upon publication. Volumes are billed only upon actual shipment. For further information please contact the publisher.

Plague and Other Yersinia Infections

Thomas Butler

International Center for Diarrhoeal Research
Dhaka, Bangladesh
Case Western Reserve University
Cleveland, Ohio

PLENUM MEDICAL BOOK COMPANY
New York and London

Library of Congress Cataloging in Publication Data

Butler, Thomas C., date–
Plague and other Yersinia infections.

(Current topics in infectious disease)
Bibliography: p.
Includes index.
1. Plague. 2. Yersinia infections. I. Title. II. Series.
RC171.B87 1983 616.9′23 83-17467
ISBN 0-306-41414-7

233 Spring Street, New York, N.Y. 10013

Plenum Medical Book Company is an imprint of Plenum Publishing Corporation

Printed in the United States of America

To

Elisabeth, Pauline, Thomas, and Thomas

Preface

During the past decade, plague infections have persisted with undiminished importance in foci of the Americas, Africa, and Asia, while infections caused by the other yersiniae were recognized only during this decade as important agents of diarrheal and appendicitislike outbreaks in Europe, North America, and Japan. The dramatic rise of plague was abetted by the military conflict in Vietnam in the latter 1960s and persisted into the 1970s. During these years more Vietnamese people probably died of plague than American servicemen died of combat injuries. In the United States during these same years, the numbers of human cases of plague increased severalfold owing to well-entrenched endemic foci in the sylvatic rodent species of the southwestern states.

In the latter 1960s, microbiologists had changed the name of the plague bacillus from *Pasteurella pestis* to *Yersinia pestis*. The other two pathogenic species, *Yersinia enterocolitica* and *Yersinia pseudotuberculosis,* were known causes of mesenteric lymphadenitis and were believed to be rare. However, there originated a strong interest in these diseases in the European countries of Sweden, Finland, Belgium, and France. Yersiniae were frequently discovered in persons with diarrhea and acute abdominal pain simulating appendicitis. This discovery sparked a worldwide surge of scientific interest in the genus *Yersinia*.

Previous writings about the yersiniae have rarely considered plague and nonplague yersiniae together. Diseases caused by these bacteria, although their epidemiological patterns and clinical pictures are very different, have some striking similarities. Both forms of *Yersinia* infection have a predilection for lymph nodes and can disseminate via the bloodstream. The different species share certain antigens and toxins and both harbor plasmids which govern virulence.

This monograph is intended for use by students, physicians, and public health workers who wish to gain a greater understanding of these diseases. The medical aspects have been stressed and an attempt made to provide balanced coverage of epidemiology, pathogenesis and clinical features, diagnosis and treatment, and control measures. The book does not try to review all recent findings on the yersiniae, because the explosion of knowledge in the past decades has created vast quantities of information. Other sources of information have been cited for the more interested readers.

My own search for an understanding of *Yersinia* infections has taken me on a personal odyssey. After seeing patients with plague for the first time in Da Nang, Vietnam in 1969, I had opportunities to study and treat more plague victims in Da Nang and Saigon, to attend the International Symposium in Saigon in 1970, to view Yersin's notebook in Nha Trang in 1974, and to teach at the University of Saigon up to 1975. Visits to Vietnam were interspersed between stretches of laboratory and experimental work in Baltimore, Cleveland, and Stockholm. In 1978 and 1979 I made field trips to Garanhuns, Brazil. Finally, since 1981 I have been in Bangladesh to work on diarrheal diseases, incidentally finding *Yersinia* species in patients with diarrhea.

THOMAS BUTLER

Dhaka, Bangladesh

Contents

1

Introduction

During the years that have elapsed since the publication of Pollitzer's classic monograph on plague in 1954,[1] several signal events have followed which have changed our understanding and concepts of this disease. First, the name of the organism was changed from *Pasteurella pestis* to *Yersinia pestis*. The newly named genus *Yersinia* was classified in the family of bacteria Enterobacteriaceae and included *Y. enterocolitica* and *Y. pseudotuberculosis,* as well as the plague bacillus. Thus, plague joined the same bacterial family as *Escherichia coli* and it became easier to think of plague as a gram-negative rod bacterial infection. There evolved concurrently a growing awareness of *Y. enterocolitica* as a pathogen capable of causing febrile gastroenteritis, as well as an acute appendicitislike syndrome.

With the military activities in Vietnam from 1965 to 1975, there was a great resurgence of plague in that country. A renaissance of interest in the disease was sparked in the minds of young American physicians who encountered the disease in Vietnamese civilians and American soldiers. Here we were given a rare glimpse of medical history by seeing this ancient disease and rediscovering its clinical drama and horrors. Thus, we witnessed people suffering the severe pain of swollen buboes. We tried to comfort patients delirious with high fever. We were humbled by the swift progression of this disease which carried healthy individuals to death within 3 days. We were shaken by the vociferous lamentations of bereaved parents. And we had to accept the conditions of misery, poor sanitation, and rat-infested housing that the patients lived in and returned to if they recovered.

Research teams from the Walter Reed Army Institute of Research and the U.S. Naval Medical Research Unit No. 2 were sent to Vietnam and their investigators advanced our knowledge of the epidemiology, pathogenesis, and treatment of plague. In October 1970 the Symposium on Plague (in Saigon) was sponsored jointly by the Public Health Department of South Vietnam and the World Health Organization. Among the participants were such notable workers as M. Bahmanyar, M. Baltazard, D. Cavanaugh, J. Marshall, H. Mollaret, J. Poland, and B. Velimirovic. The proceedings of this symposium unfortunately remain unpublished, and I shall attempt to summarize some of the significant material from the Symposium in this monograph.

Additionally, the *Journal of Infectious Diseases* planned a supplemental issue in 1973 to celebrate the 85th birthday of K. F. Meyer. By a tragic coincidence Dr. Meyer died of cancer just before its publication and it became a commemorative issue.[2] Most of the articles were concerned with immunization against plague and were written by Dr. Meyer and his associates. This issue is a fitting memorial to one of the most productive and influential workers in the field of plague since Alexandre Yersin himself. The portion of this monograph that concerns plague vaccines will summarize portions of Dr. Meyer's work and discuss some possible directions for the control of plague in the world today. A short biographical sketch of Dr. Meyer is included in Chapter 2.

Our understanding of the contributions and life of Alexandre Yersin has been greatly advanced by the recent release of the personal letters of Yersin and his niece to Dr. Mollaret. The contents of some of these letters have been published by Dr. Mollaret, who has kindly allowed me to translate selected excerpts for inclusion in this monograph. These letters should enlighten us about controversies surrounding the character of this remarkable man, who would surely be surprised to learn of the posthumous honor of having this bacterial genus named after him.

My purpose in writing this monograph is not to produce an exhaustive or comprehensive review of the *Yersinia* infections but only to discuss highlights of more recent developments in our understanding of these diseases. The larger portion of the monograph will be concerned with medical aspects of human plague and infections caused by the other *Yersinia* species. The sections will be devoted to considerations of epidemiology, pathogenesis, immunology, and therapy. I would refer the reader wishing to find recent review articles, monographs, and textbook chapters on the yersiniae to several writings that were helpful to me in approaching this subject. Helpful writings on plague after Pollitzer's monograph include writings of Bahmanyar and Cavanaugh, Brubaker, Meyer, Poland, and Reed *et al.*[3–7] Comprehensive articles on nonplague yersiniae are scarcer, but the reader may consult Nilehn, Mollaret, Bottone, and Kohl.[8–11] The International Symposium on Yersinia, 3rd, was held in Montreal, Canada, in 1977. The proceedings of this symposium were published in 1979,[12] and the 47 scientific papers in it provide a wealth of information on the epidemiology, microbiology, and pathogenesis of the nonplague yersiniae.

REFERENCES

1. R. Pollitzer, *Plague,* Monograph Series, World Health Organization, Geneva (1954).
2. *J. Infect. Dis.* **129**(Suppl.) (1974).
3. M. Bahmanyar and D. C. Cavanaugh, *Plague Manual,* World Health Organization, Geneva (1976).
4. R. R. Brubaker, The genus *Yersinia:* Biochemistry and genetics of virulence, *Curr. Topics Microbiol. Immunol.* **57:**111–158 (1972).
5. K. F. Meyer, Pneumonic plague, *Bacteriol. Rev.* **25:**249–261 (1961).
6. J. D. Poland, Plague, in *Infectious Diseases,* Second Edition (P. D. Hoeprich, ed.). Harper and Row, Hagerstown, pp. 1050–1060 (1977).
7. W. P. Reed, D. L. Palmer, R. C. Williams, and A. L. Kisch, Bubonic plague in the southwestern United States, *Medicine* **49:**465–486 (1970).
8. B. Nilehn, Studies on *Yersinia enterocolitica* with special reference to bacterial diagnosis and occurrence in human acute enteric disease, *Acta Pathol. Microbiol. Scand.* **206**(Suppl.)**:**1–48 (1969).
9. H. H. Mollaret, l'Infection humaine à *Yersinia enterocolitica* in 1970, à la lumière de 642 cas recents: Aspects cliniques et perspectives épidémiologiqes, *Pathol. Biol.* **19:**189–205 (1971).
10. E. J. Bottone, *Yersinia enterocolitica:* A panoramic view of a charismatic microorganism, *CRC Crit. Rev. Microbiol.* **5:**211–241 (1977).
11. S. Kohl, *Yersinia enterocolitica* infections, *Pediatr. Clin. North Am.* **26:**433–443 (1979).
12. P. B. Carter, L. Lafleur, and S. Toma, *Yersinia enterocolitica: Biology, Epidemiology, and Pathology, Volume 5, Contributions to Microbiology and Immunology,* S. Karger, Basel (1979).

2

Discovery of the Organisms

2.1. LIFE OF ALEXANDRE YERSIN (1863–1943)

2.1.1. Youth and Education

The discovery of the plague bacillus is credited to Alexandre Yersin, who accomplished this feat at the age of 31 years in Hong Kong in June, 1894. A chronology of the important events in Yersin's life is listed in Table 2.1.

He was born in Aubonne, Switzerland, in 1863. His father was a naturalist and widely known for his study of cockroaches. He had a sister Emilie. He was close to his mother, as his devoted twice-weekly correspondence to her from 1884 to 1905 verifies. These letters contain a wealth of exquisite detail concerning all of his travel observations, his scientific pursuits in lay terms, and his sensitive feelings. Accordingly, these letters provide important clues about the mysterious personality of this shy and introverted man, who abruptly departed a bright and promising future in medical research, in the heady last years of Pasteur's life in those stimulating laboratories, for an uncertain future of lonely travel in the steamy tropical forests of French Indochina.

Yersin began his medical studies in Lausanne, Switzerland. Then he moved to Marburg, Germany, and completed his studies in Paris, France. He became a French citizen in 1888. He chose pathology as his specialized interest because he was too shy to have close contact with patients and other physicians in the hospital setting of clinical medicine. He became interested in tuber-

TABLE 2.1
Chronology of Important Events in Yersin's Life

1863	Born in Aubonne, Switzerland
1883–1888	Medical studies in Lausanne, Switzerland; Marburg, Germany; and Paris, France
1888	Thesis on septicemic tuberculosis
1888–1890	Student of Louis Pasteur and work with Emile Roux on diphtheria toxin
1890	Departure for Indochina as ship physician for Compagnie des Messageries Maritimes
1891–1894	Geographical explorations in Vietnam and Cambodia
1892	Joined Colonial Health Corps in Saigon with Albert Calmette
1894 (June)	Isolated and described plague bacillus in Hong Kong
1895	Founded Pasteur Institute in Nha Trang, Vietnam, and lived there the rest of his life
1895–1943	Production of vaccines and antisera against plague and other infections of Indochina; work on agronomy, including importation of rubber trees and cinchona trees
1902	Founded medical school in Hanoi
1905	Death of Yersin's mother
1933	Elected member of Scientific Council of the Pasteur Institute
1933–1940	Annual visits to Paris
1940	Last visit to Paris
1943	Death in Nha Trang

culosis and in 1887 he traveled to Berlin to meet Robert Koch, the discoverer of the tubercle bacillus. His initial investigations of tuberculosis, probably stimulated by Koch, concerned the effect of antiseptics and heat on tubercle bacilli. Yersin's medical thesis was based on an experimental variety of septicemic tuberculosis.

2.1.2. Paris: Influence of Pasteur, Work with Roux on Diphtheria

While working as an assistant pathologist at the Hôtel-Dieu hospital in Paris in 1886, Yersin accidentally cut his hand during an autopsy of a patient who had died with rabies. He promptly reported to Pasteur's clinic for anti-rabies immunization. During the course of his preventive treatment he met Louis Pasteur and his assistant Emile Roux. Yersin was impressed with their work and was, of course, grateful that he survived without getting rabies. He decided to join Pasteur's group and chose to work closely with Roux on the recently discovered diphtheria bacillus.

For three years, until 1890, Yersin labored with Roux on studies of the diphtheria toxin. They co-authored three papers that would later lead the way to Roux's development of a successful immunization against diphtheria. Working together they showed that filtered cultures of growing diphtheria bacilli, free of bacteria, were capable of killing guinea pigs inoculated with 0.1 cm^3 of the filtered material within 48 hr. Pasteur's biographer, Vallery-Radot,[(7)] states that "Pasteur has long recognised the very great qualities in this pupil [Yersin], whose habits of silent labor were almost those of an ascete." It was therefore surprising that in 1890, when Yersin was in the midst of exciting scientific discoveries with Roux, he decided to leave Paris to be a ship's physician on a merchant maritime line in the Far East. Before departing (on a day Roux was absent from the laboratory) he left a long letter for Roux and for the laboratory assistants giving them instructions on how to proceed with their scientific experiments.

2.1.3. The Orient: Explorations in Indochina

Doubtless Yersin had been stimulated during his studies in Paris by teachers who had served as physicians in the colonies and had told stories of exotic travels. Although he was a small man in stature, he had great physical endurance and a strong desire for adventure and lonely hardships. Yersin's ships traveled between Manila and Saigon and Haiphong. Whenever the opportunity presented itself, Yersin disembarked his ship and made explorations of the land. He had become a geographer in realizing that the inland areas of Indochina had not been explored or mapped by any European. We can only speculate about the motives that this physician from Paris might have had to risk his life in the malarious jungles of Indochina among hostile peoples, other than curiosity and a restless courage to penetrate unknown places. In part, he may have been motivated by the French colonial drive to develop the colonies economically, in a manner similar to David Livingstone's zeal to chart the inland rivers of Africa in order to open up the continent for British trade.

Between 1891 and 1894 Yersin made several journeys of exploration in Indochina, as shown in Figure 2.1. At that time Indochina was a French colony—a loose federation that included the kingdoms of Laos and Cambodia,

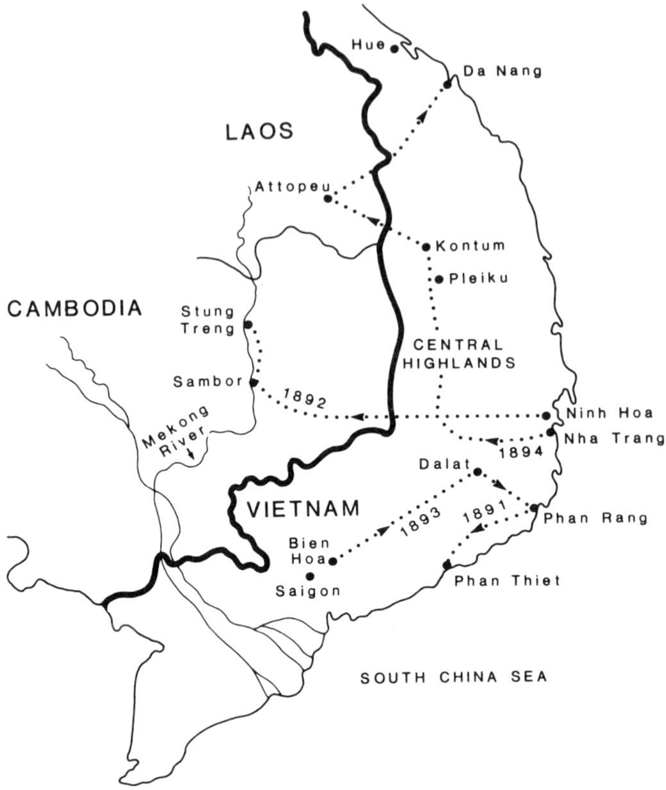

Figure 2.1. Map of Indochina showing routes of Alexandre Yersin's explorations between 1891 and 1894. Adapted from J. C. Rosenberg.[(8)]

along with the three regions of what had been and is again Vietnam: Cochin China (the southern Mekong Delta area near Saigon), Annam (the central coastal strip and inland mountains stretching from Saigon up to Northern Vietnam), and Tonkin (the northern regions around Hanoi). There were many French Catholic missionaries in Indochina seeking to convert and civilize the Vietnamese, and there was resistance by many tribes to colonization. Yersin was to meet both missionaries and hostile Vietnamese during his travels.

The value of Yersin's explorations derives not only from his extraordinary drive, purpose, and fearless zeal but also from his scientific discipline of careful observation. He carried the best instruments available at the time—chronometers, altimeters, and compasses—which allowed him to construct maps of rivers and mountains that were then unknown to the French colonialists. He kept careful notes of geographical details, facts about the flora and fauna, and other observations of people's habits, appearances, and societies. He made recommendations for road building, ore mining, and agriculture. From biographical material in French by N. Bernard and A. Badel and H. Mollaret,[2] we can get colorful glimpses of Yersin's travels: When Yersin arrived from France on the 12th of October in 1890, he immediately embarked on the "Eridan," the small boat plying between Cochin China and the Philippines, from Saigon to Manila. When this line was cut off six months later, he worked on another boat from Saigon to Haiphong. Being a fearless walker, he made quick excursions into the country whenever he was on land. From the gangway of the small boat plying along the coast of Annam, he looked with eagerness at the Annamese Chain, on which no European had ever set foot. What a wonderful adventure it would be to climb over it! By July 1891, Yersin could no longer stand the temptation. He landed in Nha Trang, intending to walk to Saigon through the mountains. The 500 km to negotiate on foot, including unforseeable obstacles, rising rivers, flooded valleys, and unreachable passes, made for a real challenge. There were travel routes; narrow paths had been made by the few inhabitants of the forest or the wild beasts in the jungle. Yersin had borrowed from the boat a chronometer and a compass. Wearing sandals and carrying five cans of corned beef in his haversack, he started off. He went southward to the small harbor of Phan Rang. A French missionary, who had several times fled from xenophobic persecution to the mountains, provided him with a guide who spoke Moi (Montagnard). A few hamlets with some huts were hidden in dense and continuous forests. In the teeming rain, the two travelers went through a pass at 900 m and arrived on the plateau of Djiring at 1200 m. Their aim was to descend from that point to Cochin China by the most direct way, but none of the inhabitants of the country agreed to guide them. The only way of escape was to return to the coast by the same route. Bare-footed, with bleeding feet, and raggedly dressed in the rain, Yersin found a junk by the seashore, which sailed him back to Nha Trang. He arrived just as his boat was going to weigh anchor for Tonkin.

Henceforth, Yersin could not free himself from the passion for travel. On the advice of Albert Calmette, who came to Saigon in 1891 to set up the first branch of the Pasteur Institute in the world and who later would be famous for developing a vaccine against tuberculosis, Yersin quit the Shipping Company to join the "Corps de Santé Colonial." On the 29th of March 1892, he departed again, on an officially authorized mission, this time to explore a region between the coast of Annam and Mekong at the level of Nha Trang.

For 3 months, he traveled without any European companions, hiring porters at each village. He traveled without benefit of landmarks. His only escorts were three young Annamese, only two of whom followed him to the end. He had only small goods for money exchange, and he was afraid that he might run short of them before the end of the journey. Sometimes he was forced to make big detours or even to retrace his route, when village chiefs would not allow him to pass. He walked in the rain or under the hot sun for 8 to 10 hr every day.

Yersin made many observations and took pictures. He discovered a tributary of the Mekong and sailed from its source to its mouth. An excerpt from his diary, dated the 16th of May, can give an idea of the difficulties encountered during this expedition:

> The storm is coming. I advance with the guide. I take with me my chronometer. The roads are bad. We find a big swamp, in which we have water up to our waist. There is an incredible quantity of leeches. My poor Mois! There, the rain is coming. The night is so dark that I cannot see my guide, even though I walk by grasping him. We go through, I think, a forest, paddy-fields (where I lose my shoes in the mud), and a bamboo forest. Finally we hear from the distance the tam-tam and the gongs. Guided by this sound, we finally arrive. Fortunately the chronometer has not been affected during this night trip.

Yersin was to make two further long journeys. The first one was from Bien Hoa to Phan Thiet, from February to October 1893, during which he discovered the Langbian Plateau. This was a beautiful spot with a temperate climate and luxuriant flowering plants. Yersin liked this plateau with its tall trees, lakes, and waterfalls so much that he recommended that a town he built as a hill station for French civil servants during vacation. Thus, the city of Dalat was founded and lovely villas were built for only the French to use. Dalat became a source of vegetables and fruits, including lettuce and strawberries, for the lowland areas of Vietnam.

A second exploration was from the coast of Annam to Darlac and Attopeu, returning through Tourane (Da Nang), from the 12th of February to the 7th of May 1894. During these travels Yersin writes that, although he had a very strong constitution, he succumbed to attacks of malaria and dysentery. Once he encountered hostile "Chinese pirates," fought them with a revolver in hand, and received a gunshot wound in his leg. At one time a tiger entered his camp and attacked a member of his group. On another occasion he witnessed the execution by Annamites of a man, who required four blows of a saber for his head to fall. Figure 2.1 shows the routes of Yersin's explorations between 1891 and 1894.

2.1.4. Discovery of the Plague Bacillus

With these grueling experiences behind him Yersin returned to Pasteurian science. In 1894 an epidemic of plague struck the Yunnan Province of China and threatened Tonkin. Yersin wanted to apply Pasteur's methods of bacteriological culture to patients with plague. He obtained permission and funding to visit Hong Kong. He arrived on June 15, 1894, with a staff of only two untrained persons, one of whom promptly absconded with Yersin's money. His only equipment was a microscope and an autoclave. In contrast, a Japanese mission headed by Shibasaburo Kitasato, a former student of Robert Koch, had arrived a few days earlier and had superior equipment and personnel. Yersin complained that the Japanese had bribed the hospital personnel not to give him facilities for autopsies. He protested to the governor of the island, who gave Yersin permission to build a straw hut on the grounds of the Alice Memorial Hospital to serve as his laboratory. Yersin actually visited Kitasato in Hong Kong, but they had no common language in which to communicate. Furthermore, their rivalry was evident by Yersin's statement "I shall avoid their society; if one of us goes off on a false track, the other will not imitate or follow him." It took Yersin only 5 days after arriving in Hong Kong to isolate the organism in culture, and in the incredibly short period of 7 weeks, he made brilliant observations on the epidemiology, clinical features, pathology, bacteriology, experimental infections, and immunology that are incisively described in his paper[1] that was published in the same year. The following is a translation of a letter to Yersin's mother that he wrote 9 days after arriving in Hong Kong*:

Hong Kong
June 24, 1894

Dear Mother,

I am certain that you must be a little anxious to receive this letter, as I am aware that I am in a place where one doesn't exactly go for a pleasure trip!

After having stayed at the hotel for some days, I have built myself a straw hut near the hospital for the plague victims and there I have set up my living quarters and my laboratory.

All that did not happen without difficulty, and if I would not have had the good fortune to meet a fine Catholic missionary who was willing to accompany me everywhere and to serve as my interpreter, I don't know how I would have managed. The missionary's name is Father Vigano. He has lived in Hong Kong for thirty years and knows everybody.

* Translated from the French[2] by Ingrid Ebner with permission of H. H. Mollaret.

> The Japanese have sent a commission to study the plague too. This commission is composed of six members. They arrived a few days before I did and they believe themselves to be the only ones to have the right to study the disease! In order to stop me from doing anything, they have bribed the staff of the hospital so that they will not provide me with an autopsy! I have complained to the governor and today I have the same working conditions as they.
>
> I have already studied a dozen cases, and it has not been difficult for me to discover the microbe which swarms in the buboes, in the lymph nodes, in the spleen, etc. This is a little rod, a little longer than it is wide and which can be dyed easily. It kills mice, guinea pigs with the lesions of the plague. I will find it again, there isn't any doubt.
>
> With this post [mail] I am sending to the Pasteur Institute a certain number of small sealed tubes containing pulp of the plague bubo. Then the study of the disease can begin in Paris. Here I am very limited in my experiments because my laboratory is very poorly equipped.
>
> Hong Kong is a very picturesque city, built on the shore of the sea on the side of a steep mountain of 600 meters. The houses are ranged in tiers up to the top. The Chinese population numbers 200,000 souls. Today it is reduced to half on account of the emigration brought on by the plague. We are in the middle of the rainy season, it rains a downright deluge of water and following each of these violent downpours we have an increase of the epidemic.
>
> Mortality is very high, 95% of the cases. Up to the present only three Englishmen have been stricken. I don't count the Portuguese, there are so many. One of these days I shall try to make a small photograph of my straw hut with me in front of it, and I shall send it to you.
>
> I continue to do very well, only a little tired, because I am alone I have to do everything.
>
> As servants I have an Indo-Chinese boy who has accompanied me on my last trip to the Mois (an aboriginal mountain tribe) and a Chinese boy whom the Father has got for me as replacement for another whom I had recruited at Haiphong and who disappeared the other day having stolen 80 piastras from me.
>
> I eat either at the English club with the French Consul or at home, because the hospital for the plague victims is half an hour from the center of town by rickshaw.
>
> I still have many things to tell you, but there are two cadavers waiting for me and these gentlemen are in a great hurry, it seems, to go to the cemetery. Farewell, dear mother, wash your hands after having read my letter so that you won't catch the plague!!
>
> Your affectionate son,
>
> Dr. Yersin

It must be remarked that this letter, as well as numerous others written by Yersin to his mother, was composed in a lucid journalistic style that contained no personal news for his mother nor suggested that his mother was answering any of this series of letters. Rather the letters appeared to be documents that Yersin intended to be preserved as a record of his life. The impersonal, one-way quality of this correspondence is also exemplified by his formal signature "Dr. Yersin."

The following are translated excerpts from Yersin's classic paper of 1894[6]:

> At the beginning of last May there erupted in Hong Kong an epidemic of bubonic plague which was taking a heavy toll of the population. The disease had been endemic for a very long time on the high plateau of Yunnan, and had appeared from time to time very close to the border of our Indochinese territories, in Mong-Tse, Lang-Tcheou and Pakhoi. In March, this year, plague appeared in Canton and in a few weeks caused the death of 60,000 persons in the city alone. The great commercial traffic which exists between Canton and Hong Kong and also between Hong Kong and Tonkin has worried the French authorities that Indochina might be struck by the epidemic. This fear is well founded since it is difficult to establish an efficacious quarantine in these regions.
>
> I received from the Ministry of Colonies the order to go to Hong Kong to study the nature of this affliction, the conditions under which it spreads, and the methods to curb it, in order to prevent its reaching our territories.
>
> When I arrived in that city, the 15th of June, more than 300 Chinese had already died. As rapidly as possible, temporary structures were erected, since the hospitals of the colony were overflowing.
>
> I settled with my laboratory equipment in a straw hut that I had built with the permission of the English government, on the grounds of the main hospital.
>
> The disease, which was almost exclusively in the Chinese boroughs of the city, had all the symptoms and all the characteristics of the ancient bubonic plague which, in past centuries, had decimated many times the populations of occidental Europe as well as those of the East. The famous epidemic of Marseille, in 1720, was the last one that affected France. Since that time the plague has been limited to a few foci in Persia and Arabia and in the Chinese province of Yunnan.
>
> Here are the symptoms of the disease:
>
> The onset is rapid, with an incubation period of $4\frac{1}{2}$ to 6 days. The patient is prostrated.
>
> Abruptly a high fever sets in, often accompanied by delirium. On the very first day a discrete bubo usually appears. In 75% of the cases it is located in the inguinal region, in 10% of the cases in the axillary region, and occasionally at the back of the neck or in other regions.
>
> The nodule rapidly reaches the size of an egg. Death occurs after 48 hours and often sooner. If the patient manages to survive 5 to 6 days, the prognosis is better, the bubo softens and one can operate to drain the pus.
>
> In a few cases, the bubo does not have the time to form, and one will note in such cases hemorrhages in the mucous membranes or petechial spots on the skin.
>
> Mortality is high; 95% in the hospitals.
>
> In the infected boroughs, many dead rats are found on the ground. It is interesting to note that in the part of the town where the epidemic started, a new sewage duct has just been installed. The pipes are much too narrow and are difficult to clean. They constitute a permanent focus of infection. One does not understand why there are two different sewage networks in Hong Kong. One is narrow and chronically clogged and is used for the disposal of water from the

houses. The other is large and well planned, and is used for the disposal of rain water.

The toilets are mobile and are emptied every day; the contents are used, after a certain amount of treatment, as fertilizer for the innumerable gardens which border the Canton River opposite the island of Hong Kong.

The lodging quarters of the poor Chinese are often so revoltingly dirty that one scarcely has the courage to enter them. In addition, the number of occupants is unbelievable. Many of these slums do not have windows and are below the level of the ground. One can imagine the havoc that can be caused by an epidemic on such a terrain and the difficulty involved in its control. The only remedy was to burn down the Chinese town. This was proposed but was unfeasible for budgetary reasons.

Few Europeans have been struck by the disease, thanks to the better conditions under which they live. European houses are not fully safe, however, since even there one can encounter dead rats.

The physicians of the Chinese Customs, who had the occasion to observe the epidemics of Pakhoi and Lien-Chu, in the province of Canton, and Mr. Rocher, French Consul in Mong-Tse, had remarked that the scourge starts by severely affecting mice, buffaloes, and pigs before striking men. . . .

The fact that certain animals were naturally susceptible to the disease gave me the proper material for its experimental study.

It seemed logical to start first by looking for a microbe in the blood of patients and in the pulp of the buboes. The pulp of the buboes always contains masses of short, stubby bacilli which are rather easy to stain with aniline dyes and are not stained by the method of Gram. The ends of the bacilli are colored more strongly than the center. Sometimes the bacilli seem to be surrounded by a capsule. One can find them in large numbers in the buboes and the lymph nodes of the diseased persons. They are seen in the blood from time to time, but less abundantly than in the buboes and lymph nodes, and only in very serious and rapidly fatal cases.

The pulp of buboes, seeded on agar, gives rise to transparent, white colonies with margins that are iridescent when examined with reflected light.

Growth is even better if glycerol is incorporated into the agar. The bacillus also grows on coagulated serum.

In broth, the bacillus has a very characteristic appearance resembling that of the erysipelas culture: clear liquid with lumps depositing on the walls and bottom of the tube.

The most favorable medium is an alkaline solution of 2% peptone to which 1 to 2% gelatine has been added.

Microscopical examination of the cultures reveals true chains of short bacilli interspersed with larger spherical bodies. . . . As the cultures get older, swollen and abnormal forms become more common, and these do not stain easily. [See Figure 2.2B.]

If one inoculates mice, rats, or guinea pigs with the pulp from buboes, they die, and at autopsy one can note the characteristic lesions as well as numerous bacilli in the lymph nodes, spleen, and blood. Guinea pigs die in 2 to 5 days, mice in 1 to 3 days. In the first passages, the microbes are mainly in the mononuclear leukocytes.

In the guinea pig after a few hours one can already detect edema at the point of inoculation and the surrounding lymph nodes become palpable. After 24 hours, the hair of the guinea pig is ruffled, it will no longer eat, and it is suddenly seized by convulsive crises which become more and more frequent until death.

At autopsy there are hemorrhages in the abdominal cavity. The site of inoculation is edematous and the edema extends to the regional lymph node, which is enlarged and full of bacilli. The intestine is often hyperemic. The adrenal capsules are congested, the kidneys are violaceous, and the liver is enlarged and red. The spleen is also enlarged and often covered with an eruption of small miliary tubercles. When the disease has lasted somewhat longer than usual, there are sometimes abscesses in the abdominal wall.

In the pleura and peritoneum, there is a small amount of serous liquid that contains the bacillus. The organism can also be found in the blood, where it is more elongated than in the lymph nodes. The liver and the spleen are also very rich in microbes.

Passages in guinea pigs are easily achieved with macerated spleen or blood. Death is more rapid after a few passages.

Pigeons do not die after having been inoculated with a moderate dose of either the pulp of the bubo or the culture of the plague bacillus.

The first culture from a bubo is difficult to establish on peptone agar. It grows, however, and kills as fast as the pulp of the bubo.

One notes, after a few days, that in these cultures certain colonies grow faster than others. Examined with the microscope, they all contain the pure bacillus. . . . If one inoculates the faster growing strains into animals one notes that their virulence is strongly diminished. They kill the guinea pigs only after a rather long time or they do not kill them at all, but they are still fatal for white mice.

I have noted that on agar the less virulent colonies grow faster than the others and tend to predominate. The net result is that upon successive transfers the cultures rapidly lose virulence.

One can often kill mice, and almost always rats, by feeding them fragments of spleen or liver from animals which have died of plague. At autopsy, one recovers the bacillus from the blood, the liver, the spleen, and the lymph nodes.

The mice that have survived many contaminated meals die when they are injected subcutaneously.

Dead rats that one finds in houses and in the streets almost always harbor large quantities of the microbe in their organs. Many have real buboes.

I have placed healthy mice and inoculated mice in the same cage. The inoculated ones died first, but within a few days, all the others die of invasion with the plague bacillus.

Plague is thus a contagious and transmissible disease. It is probable that the rats are the major vector of its propagation, but I have also noted that flies can acquire the disease and die. Thus flies may also be an agent in its transmission.

I had noted that there were many dead flies in the laboratory where I was performing my autopsies. The body of a fly was freed of wings, and the legs and head ground in broth and inoculated into a guinea pig. The inoculum contained a large number of bacilli which were similar to the plague organism and the guinea pig died in 48 hours with the specific lesions of the disease.

I have been able to isolate the plague bacillus from soil which had been collected 4 to 5 centimeters under the surface in a house where disinfection efforts

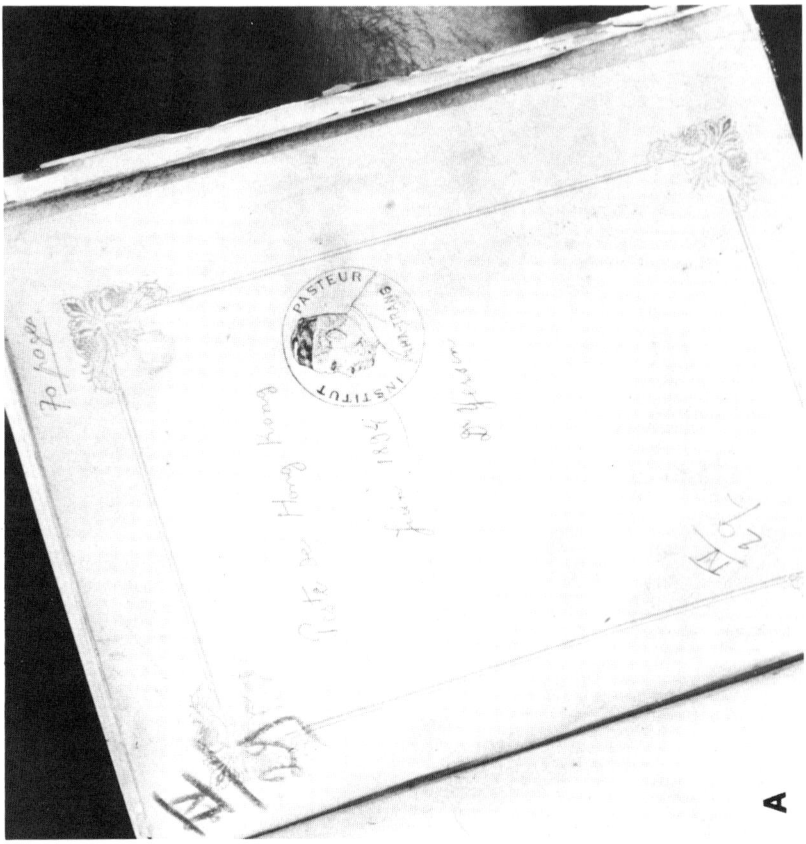

A

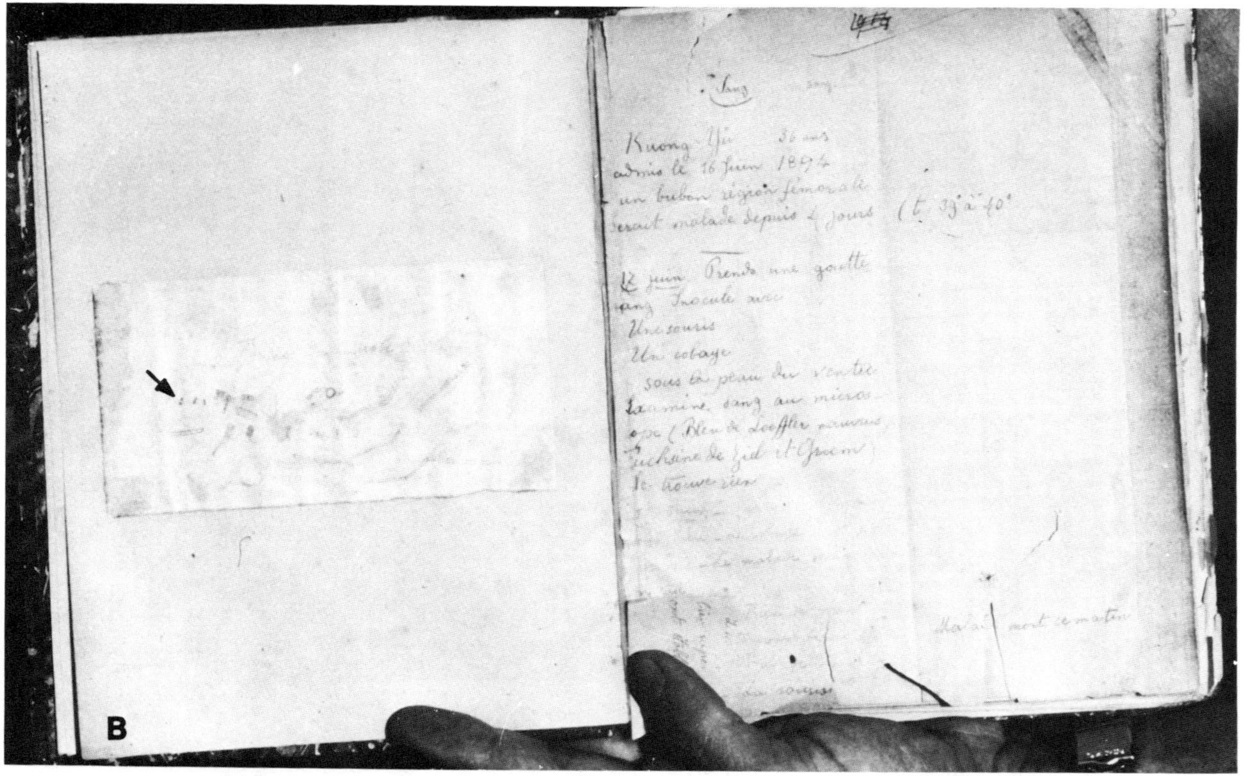

Figure 2.2. The notebook of Yersin's on plague in Hong Kong that is displayed at the Pasteur Institute in Nha Trang, Vietnam. (A) The title page of the journal. (B) Pages that include Yersin's drawing of the microscopical appearance of the plague bacillus. The arrow points to the short bipolar form. On the other page are notes about a patient with plague.

had been made. It was in all respects similar to the one isolated from buboes, but it was not virulent.

I have mentioned previously that in cultures from blood or from a bubo one could isolate several varieties of the bacillus which differed in their virulence to animals, and that some colonies had even lost all virulence for the guinea pig. From a bubo of a patient who had recovered and had been convalescing for three weeks, I was able to isolate a few colonies which completely lacked virulence to mice. . . .

These very telling facts permit me to suppose that the inoculation of certain strains or varieties with little or no virulence would be able to give animals immunity against plague. I have started some experiments in this direction and I shall publish their results in the future.

The notebook that Yersin used in Hong Kong is on public display in Nha Trang. Figure 2.2 shows selected pages of that notebook, including Yersin's own original drawing of the microscopical forms of the bacteria.

Yersin returned to Paris in October 1894 to present his results to his teacher Roux. Pasteur, at the age of 72, was in the last year of his life and gained great satisfaction from reading Yersin's account of applying his own methods to elucidate the cause of plague. Conferring with Roux, Yersin made plans to make an attenuated live vaccine and an antiserum to be used for the prevention and treatment of plague. The following year Yersin returned to Indochina and founded the Pasteur Institute at Nha Trang for the production of vaccines and antisera.

2.1.5. The Yersin–Kitasato Controversy

Since June 1894 there has been much discussion and disagreement over who should be credited with the discovery of the plague bacillus or whether Yersin and Kitasato should be co-discoverers.

Kitasato arrived in Hong Kong on June 12, 1894 (3 days before Yersin) and established himself at the Kennedy Town Hospital. Like Yersin, he promptly reported his results the same year.[(3)] On June 14, 1894, he observed an autopsy of a plague victim and found bacilli in the bubo, blood, lungs, liver, and spleen. He noted the bipolar staining with aniline dyes. He prepared broth cultures and inoculated mice and other animals which died with the same bacilli present in their organs. These first reports of Yersin and Kitasato[(1,3)] are remarkably similar in several respects, including similar descriptions of the virulence of the bacilli for laboratory animals (but not for pigeons!), the virulence for animals fed pieces of infected organs, and the isolation of bacilli from the soil of Hong Kong. Furthermore, both investigators carefully described the bipolar nature of the bacilli when they were stained with aniline dyes, leaving little doubt that Yersin and Kitasato had both correctly recognized the causative agent of plague. The differences between their initial descriptions were relatively minor, as shown in Table 2.2. Only Yersin correctly described the gram-negative nature of the bacillus and its tendency to form lumps or flocculent stands in broth. Kitasato apparently erred in describing the organism as slightly motile and having an optimal growth temperature ranging higher than 30°C, but Yersin did not attempt to describe these features at all.

In the aftermath of these signal reports on the bacterial cause of plague, there was a series of confusing statements and self-contradictions by Kitasato and his colleagues that tended to discredit his claim to have been the codiscoverer of the plague bacillus.[4,5] The cultures and subcultures of human blood that Kitasato subsequently worked with were reported to be gram-positive and to resemble pneumococci. These cultures might have, in fact, been contaminated by the pneumococcus. Thus, he asserted that his and Yersin's bacilli were different. Later, however, he changed his views to be that both bacilli were the same, representing merely variant forms of each other.

TABLE 2.2
Differences between Yersin's and Kitasato's Original Descriptions of the Plague Bacillus in 1894 and the Modern Concept of the Bacterium *Yersinia pestis*

	Gram stain reaction	Motility	Appearance in broth	Optimal growth temperature
Yersin	Gram-negative	Not mentioned	Clear liquid lumps depositing on the walls and bottom of the tube	Not mentioned
Kitasato	Unable to say whether method can be employed	Slightly motile	Somewhat cloudy	26–39°C
Modern	Gram-negative	Nonmotile	Flocculent strands	25–30°C

The origins and reasons for the controversy over whether Yersin or Kitasato was the first to recognize and culture the plague bacillus have been recently reviewed by Howard-Jones[4] and Bibel and Chen.[5] Whatever the correct interpretation of events is, Yersin emerges as the better bacteriologist for several reasons:

1. Yersin's original description had the correct gram stain reaction and did not contain errors.
2. Yersin's cultures were pure, whereas Kitasato's probably were contaminated with the pneumococcus.
3. After Kitasato left Hong Kong, he was busy starting a large laboratory in Japan and allowed himself and colleagues to issue false claims and self-contradictory statements.
4. Yersin went to Paris to confer with Roux, who verified the nature of Yersin's bacillus and directed Yersin to develop an antiserum to treat patients with plague.

2.1.6. Further Work on Plague

Yersin returned to Vietnam in 1895 to establish the Pasteur Institute in Nha Trang for the purpose of producing plague antiserum in horses. He experimented with this antisera in patients in Nha Trang. In 1896 plague was still rife in China and he visited Hong Kong again, as well as Canton and Amoy, to use his revolutionary treatment in plague victims. An epidemic of plague broke out in India in May 1897 and Yersin introduced his antiserum in Bombay and Mandvi.

2.1.7. Other Activities

Yersin was a man of manifold talents and diversified drives. He settled into a house in Nha Trang, which he equipped with the accessories of his hobbies, including cameras, telescopes, radios, and a telegraph. He became interested in tropical agronomy. He imported Brazilian rubber trees and cinchona trees, which he labored to acclimate to Indochina at the right altitude and climate. He became interested in animal diseases and introduced new prophylaxes and treatments for veterinary diseases, especially in horses, cows, and buffaloes. Twenty kilometers north of Nha Trang he developed a plantation for farming and raising animals near the river Suoi Giao.

In 1902, General Governor Paul Doumer invited Yersin to Hanoi for a discussion on the establishment of a medical school, of which Yersin would be the director. He accepted. By the end of 1904, he had been replaced and went back to Nha Trang. He became the director of two laboratories in Saigon and Nha Trang, which then were changed formally into Pasteur Institutes with the name "Pasteur Institutes in Indochina."

2.1.8. Final Years

In 1933 Yersin was elected a member of the Scientific Council of the Pasteur Institute. He dutifully fulfilled this task by making annual visits to Paris to attend the Council's meetings. His last visit to Paris was in 1940 at the outbreak of World War II. Allegedly, he married a Montagnard woman, with whom he lived in Nha Trang, but he had no children. He preferred to complete his life in the lonely exile of Indochina than to return to Europe. He remained a shy man who avoided going to meetings and who valued solitude above all else. When he died in 1943 he was buried, according to his will, on the plantation he had developed near the Suoi Giao River. The appreciation of the Vietnamese people for Yersin's service to their country was shown by the naming of streets of Vietnamese cities after him. The Pasteur Institute on the bay at Nha Trang was still functioning in 1975 to make vaccines and sera, and his home on the laboratory grounds beside the beach has been preserved as a museum with his scientific notebooks, library, and photographic and astronomic devices on display for visitors.

2.2. NOMENCLATURE

The plague bacillus was initially known as *Bacterium pestis* until 1900, when it was renamed *Bacillus pestis*. After 1923 it was called *Pasteurella pestis*. The genus *Yersinia* was first proposed by van Lognem in 1944, and in 1954 Thal suggested that this genus be included in the family Enterobacteriaceae. Only in the last decade, however, have most workers and authors finally accepted this reclassification and ceased to include the plague bacillus in the genus *Pasteurella*.

2.3. HISTORY OF *YERSINIA ENTEROCOLITICA* AND *YERSINIA PSEUDOTUBERCULOSIS*

The discovery and recognition of these other two members of the genus *Yersinia* were not attended by the same excitement and drama as the discovery of *Y. pestis,* and Yersin certainly had nothing to do with characterizing these species. Human infection by *Y. enterocolitica* was first reported in 1939 by Schleifstein and Coleman. It was then called *Bacterium enterocoliticum* but was renamed *Pasteurella X* by Daniels and Goudzwaard in 1963 and finally was grouped in the genus *Yersinia* by Frederiksen in 1964.

Pfeiffer in 1889 first described *Bacillus pseudotuberculosis,* which he renamed *Pasteurella pseudotuberculosis* in 1929. Additionally, it was called *Shigella pseudotuberculosis* in 1935 until Smith and Thal placed it into the genus *Yersinia* in 1965.

2.4. THE LIFE AND WORK OF K. F. MEYER (1884–1974)

After the discovery of the plague bacillus by Yersin, the work of K. F. Meyer did much to advance our knowledge of plague and to stimulate the interest of other workers in this disease. Summaries of his energetic, productive, and lengthy career have been written by Steele[9] and Cavanaugh.[10]

Meyer was born in Basel, Switzerland, in 1884. He received his education at the Universities of Basel and Zurich in the fields of zoology and histology. He chose veterinary medicine and became particularly interested in infectious diseases of animals. He went to South Africa in 1910 to study animal diseases. He carried out studies of pleuropneumonia in horses and mules. He contracted malaria and returned to Switzerland for convalescence. Then he emigrated to the United States and became a Professor of Veterinary Medicine at the University of Pennsylvania in 1911. In 1913 he moved to the University of California at Berkeley. A full professor at the age of 30, he became during the next 40 years a leading investigator of several infectious diseases of both veterinary and human public health concern. These diseases, which Dr. Meyer enthusiastically undertook to study, included botulism, influenza, pseudotuberculosis, anthrax, brucellosis, tetanus, sporotrichosis, and psittacosis.

Plague captured his attention in 1920 when he began studies of sylvatic plague in rodents. The start of World War II caused Meyer to concentrate even more attention on plague research and the development of vaccines to control this infection that had potential military importance. His experimental animal studies of protection led to the usage of the present U.S.P. vaccine for plague. His work in animals was also instrumental in defining effective antibiotics for the treatment of plague.

Certain parallels between the lives of Yersin and Meyer and their important contributions to plague research are interesting. Both men were born in Switzerland in the latter half of the 19th century. Both men received parts of their scientific educations in Switzerland and then emigrated and developed interests in tropical medicine abroad—Yersin in Asia and Meyer in South Africa. Both men lived most of their years outside of Switzerland. Large parts of their investigative careers were spent on diseases of animals not limited to plague infection, and the wide-ranging diversity of diseases that both men undertook to control contrasts sharply with modern trends toward narrow specialization. The ambitious work programs and productivity of both men, especially Meyer, were legendary. Hobbies were also characteristic of these eminent men: Yersin's interests included telescopes and cameras, while Meyer collected stamps commemorating scientists. Finally, both men were blessed with native intelligence combined with infinite curiosity and courageous, boundless, adventurous drives which carried them physically over great distances as well as scientifically into new areas of knowledge. The striking differences between the two men lay in their personalities: Meyer was an extroverted and gregarious man who displayed his brilliance and enthusiasm as a great teacher and writer; Yersin was an introverted man with a desire for solitude who did relatively little teaching and writing.

REFERENCES

1. A. Yersin, La peste bubonique á Hong Kong, *Ann. Inst. Pasteur Paris* **8:**662–667 (1894).
2. H. H. Mollaret, Alexandre Yersin tel qu'en lui-même enfin . . . les révélations d'une correspondence inédite échelonée de 1884 ci 1926, *Nouv. Presse Med.* **39:**2575–2580 (1973).
3. S. Kitasato, The bacillus of bubonic plague, *Lancet* **2:**428–430 (1894).
4. N. Howard-Jones, Kitasato, Yersin and the plague bacillus, *Clio Med.* **10:**23–27 (1975).
5. D. J. Bibel and T. H. Chen, Diagnosis of plague: An analysis of the Yersin–Kitasato controversy, *Bacteriol. Rev.* **40:**633–651 (1976).
6. H. A. Lechevalier and M. Solotorovsky, *Three Centuries of Microbiology.* McGraw-Hill, New York, pp. 150–157 (1965).
7. R. Vallery-Radot, *The Life of Pasteur,* Doubleday, Page, Garden City, p. 457 (1924).
8. J. C. Rosenberg, *Doctors Afield: Alexandre Yersin, N. Engl. J. Med.* **278:**261–263 (1968).
9. J. H. Steele, Karl Friedrich Meyer, *J. Infect. Dis.* **129:**53–59 (1974).
10. D. C. Cavanaugh, K. F. Meyer's work on plague, *J. Infect. Dis.* **129:**S10–S12 (1974).

3

Epidemiology

3.1. PLAGUE

3.1.1. Cycles of Transmission

Plague is a zoonotic infection, caused by the bacterium *Yersinia pestis*. It is transmitted among the natural animal reservoirs, which are predominantly urban and sylvatic rodents (i.e., living in cities or the country), through vector flea bites or ingestion of contaminated animal tissues by the host. The cycle of infection is shown schematically in Figure 3.1. Throughout the world, the urban and domestic rats, *Rattus rattus* and *Rattus norvegicus,* are the most important reservoirs of the plague bacillus. Sylvatic plague is present in the United States, and examples of the variety of wild rodent reservoirs are itemized in Figure 3.1. Man is an accidental host in the natural cycle of plague, when he is bitten by an infected rodent flea, and appears to play no role in the maintenance of *Y. pestis* in nature. Only rarely, during epidemics of pneumonic plague, is the infection believed to be passed directly from man to man. Also rarely, man can develop infection by the direct handling of contaminated animal tissues.

The occurrence of human plague is nearly always linked to the transmission of plague among the natural animal reservoirs. The incidence of plague in humans for any particular locality is, therefore, a function of both the frequency of infection in local rodent populations and the intimacy with which the people live with the infected rodents and their fleas.

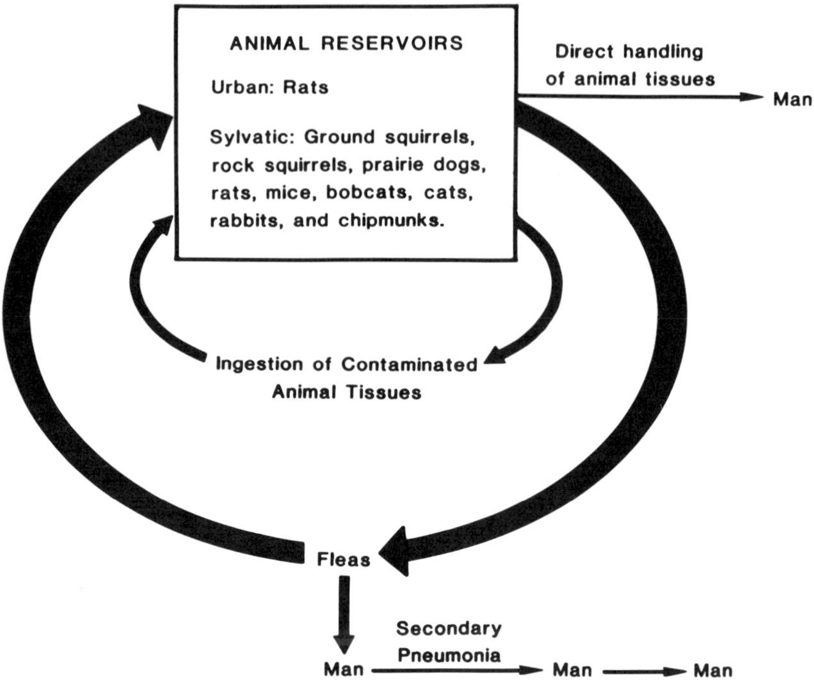

Figure 3.1. The transmission of *Yersinia pestis* among animal reservoirs and to man. Thick arrows, usual routes; medium arrows, occasional routes; thin arrows, rare routes.

3.1.2. World Distribution of Human Plague

Despite the efforts of public health workers to control plague, this infection is present in all of the major continental areas of the world. During the decade 1970–1979, human cases of plague were reported in the countries shown in Figure 3.2. This widespread distribution of human plague indicates that the infection is firmly entrenched in the world's rodent populations.[1]

A more detailed quantitative listing of the human cases of plague reported to the World Health Organization is provided in Table 3.1. The accuracy of these reported figures is, of course, severely limited by under- and overreporting. Additionally, there were no uniform criteria for defining a confirmed or suspected case. Few of these countries have modern bacteriological facilities near the endemic areas to assist physicians in making a diagnosis either

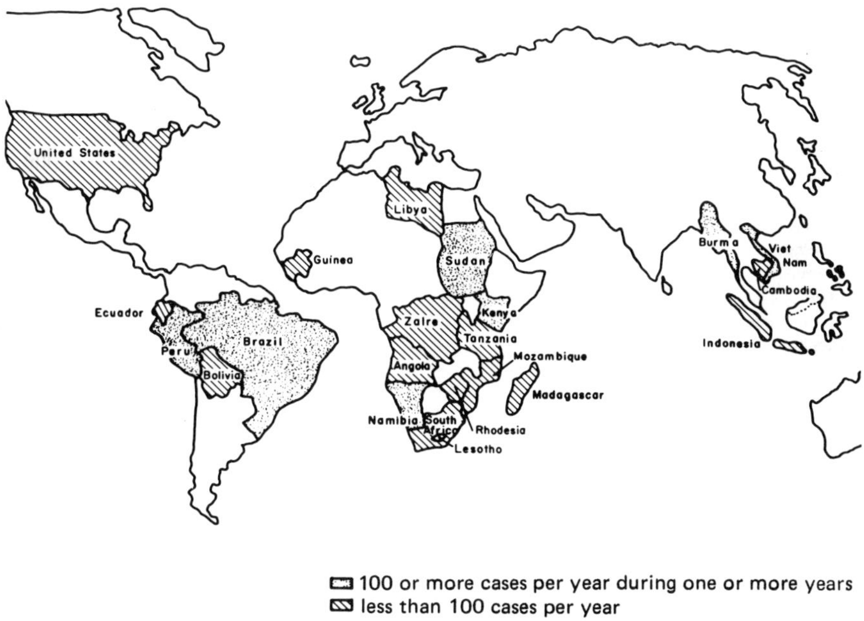

Figure 3.2. Human plague in the world from 1970 to 1979 by reporting on individual countries to the World Health Organization.

by the isolation of *Y. pestis* or by examination of paired sera for specific antibody titers. Thus, because of the inaccuracies of the data in Table 3.1, only a crude estimate of the actual incidence of plague today in the world can be made.

We are presently experiencing the fourth great pandemic in the world. The first three are believed to have occurred in the following times[(2)]: (1) the first originated in Egypt in 542 A.D. and spread to Turkey and Europe, (2) the second pandemic started in the 14th century in Asia Minor and Africa and after spreading to Europe killed about a fourth of that continent's people, and (3) the third also occurred in Europe, during the 15th to 18th centuries. The present fourth pandemic began around 1860 in the Chinese province of Yunnan. It spread to the southern coast of China reaching Hong Kong in 1894, when Yersin and Kitasato went to discover the causative bacterium. Subsequently plague was carried by ship to India and other countries of Asia, to Brazil, and to California.

TABLE 3.1
Number of Cases of Human Plague Reported to the World Health Organization during the Decade 1970–1979[a]

	1970	1971	1972	1973	1974	1975	1976	1977	1978	1979
Africa										
Angola	0	0	0	0	0	49	0	0	0	0
Guinea	3	0	0	0	0	0	0	0	0	0
Kenya	0	0	0	0	0	0	0	0	166	227
Lesotho	0	0	8	0	0	8	0	0	0	0
Libya	0	0	16	0	0	0	19	11	0	0
Madagascar	8	17	63	20	0	52	50	27	24	17
Mozambique	0	0	0	0	37	0	15	97	12	0
Namibia	0	0	0	0	102	0	0	0	0	0
South Africa	0	0	1	0	0	0	0	0	0	0
Rhodesia	0	0	0	0	23	34	0	0	0	0
Sudan	0	0	0	0	0	0	0	0	0	226
Tanzania	0	0	32	0	0	0	0	2	0	0
Zaire	16	3	8	30	20	1	12	4	0	1
TOTAL	27	20	128	50	182	144	96	141	202	471
Americas										
Bolivia	54	19	0	0	14	2	24	29	68	10
Brazil	101	146	169	152	291	496	97	1	11	0
Equador	30	27	9	1	0	0	8	0	0	0
Peru	128	22	118	30	8	3	1	0	6	0
U.S.	13	2	1	2	8	20	16	18	12	13
TOTAL	326	216	297	185	321	521	146	48	97	23
Asia										
Burma	43	189	63	17	700	275	673	591	171	73
China	0	0	0	0	0	0	0	0	0	8
Indonesia	10	0	0	0	0	0	0	0	0	0
Kampuchea	—	—	5	1	0	0	0	0	0	0
Vietnam	4056	3997	1340	425	1552	536	593	667	314	306
TOTAL	4109	4186	1408	443	2252	811	1266	1258	485	379
World TOTAL	4462	4422	1833	678	2755	1476	1508	1447	784	881

[a] Individual countries reporting larger numbers of cases are selectively included. Adapted from the *Weekly Epidemiological Record*.[1]

3.1.3. Plague in Vietnam

3.1.3.1. A Brief Historical Summary

During the 10 years of U.S. involvement in the military conflict in Vietnam, there was a great recrudescence of plague with peak numbers of 4194 cases and 216 deaths reported in 1968. Considerable efforts were made by the Walter Reed Army Institute of Research and by the World Health Organization to study the epidemiology of plague in Vietnam. Marshall, Cavanaugh, and their colleagues at the Walter Reed Army Institute of Research worked effectively to define the geographic distribution, reservoirs, and vectors of plague in Vietnam,[3–5] and Dr. Velimirovic of the World Health Organization has reviewed our present knowledge of the epidemiology of plague in southeast Asia.[6,7]

Because of the importance of Vietnam as the leading country of the world in the incidence of plague during the last decade, I will include passages of Velimirovic's historical summary, which places the current outbreaks in their historical context[6]:

> The first outbreak of plague was recorded in Nha Trang in 1898, presumably introduced from Hong Kong by shipping routes. In 1904 one case of pneumonic plague occurred on a ship with Chinese immigrants from Hong Kong. The first cases in Saigon were found in 1906 in two Indian subjects, both in immigrant quarters next to the Immigration Service. Epidemiological investigation incriminated the importation of rats in bales originating from Canton, which was infected at that time. However, the first known epidemic was initiated by a student from the Hanoi School of Medicine, who stayed a few days in Cholon* before joining his family in Bentre, where he died after starting an infection in seven persons out of whom five died. Three months later, in January 1907, plague appeared again in Saigon–Cholon, and Giadinh in April in Soctrang (now Ba Xuyen province). In 1908 a big epidemic occurred in Phan Thiet (now Ninh Thuan) province, in 1909 in Saigon–Cholon and Giadinh and in 1910 again in Scotrang imported by a sampan, and also in Phanri and Da Nang.
>
> This outbreak was characterized by a large number of septicaemic cases. In 1911 another big epidemic with pulmonary complications occurred in Giadinh, Chaudoc, Long Xuyen, Thudaumot, Soctrang and Saigon–Cholon. Plague occurred in the same provinces every year with small epidemics and occasional pneumonic cases. In addition, the disease continued to spread towards the North. In 1913 parts of Phan Rang and Ninh Tuan provinces were affected and in 1914 the provinces of Quang Nam and Vinh Long. Official records state that notified cases were only part of the totals. In 1917 plague became established in the province of Tayninh and Bienhoa. The disease continued in 1918, 1919, 1920, and 1921. Usually the same villages were affected and in Saigon–Cholon, the same parts of the town. Large scale vaccination with Haffkine vaccine was initiated in 1918. In 1920, for the first time, no cases were reported in vaccinated persons. A systematic examination of all deaths has been attempted, but *Yersinia pestis* was found only in 29 of 100 deaths clinically suspected as plague. In 1921 a surveillance system for rodent epizootics was instituted. The epidemiological work encountered many difficulties due to fear and ignorance and especially from quarantine measures which caused economic loss to the population. Dead bodies were deposited overnight in various places of the town, making tracing of the cases impossible. Strict quarantine measures were applied to all incoming ships, especially those from Hong Kong. Regular vaccination was practiced around infected cases, in addition often the infected houses were burned. Straw-roofed houses were forbidden. From 1923 to 1931 plague gradually declined. During the 1940s,

*Cholon is today a part of Saigon. At that time, it was a nearby twin city to Saigon.

plague increased but surveillance activities were difficult to maintain during the Japanese occupation and in the following years. Epidemic outbreaks were noted in 1941 in Chaudoc province (pneumonic), in 1942 and 1943 in Saigon, Phan Thiet and Phan Rang (Ninh Thuan and Binh Thuan provinces), and in 1948 in Phan Thiet (Ninh Thuan province in which plague was present continuously over 60 years). From 1942 on, plague spread to the hill country, Long Bian plateau west of Phan Rang. During the period 1952–1962 small outbreaks were reported from Saigon–Phan Thiet areas and the adjoining provinces and in 1956 from Tay Ninh with about 50 deaths.

Although many parts of the country have not been accessible to systematic surveys, it has become apparent that from 1962, massive spread of plague occurred in areas which had not been considered endemic in the earlier years. In 1965 and 1966, plague was found in almost all provinces without firm evidence of foci except the towns. [Figure 3.3.] Adequate data about the distribution of plague in the provinces are not available as all medical personnel were in the towns or in the army. Although considerable work has been done, the war situation has influenced the pattern of reporting. The surveillance improved in succeeding years, as the medical profession became thoroughly alert to the disease. Thus, for example, the first patient observed in the 1962 epidemic wave in Bien Hoa, a child of eight years, visited three hospitals and was suspected of having appendicitis or strangulated hernia and died while awaiting surgery. Postmortem and subsequent bacteriology confirmed plague. The next three confirmed cases came from a densely populated regroupment centre for refugees from North Viet Nam, composed of about 18 hamlets with thatched huts. In the years 1965/66, throat swabs

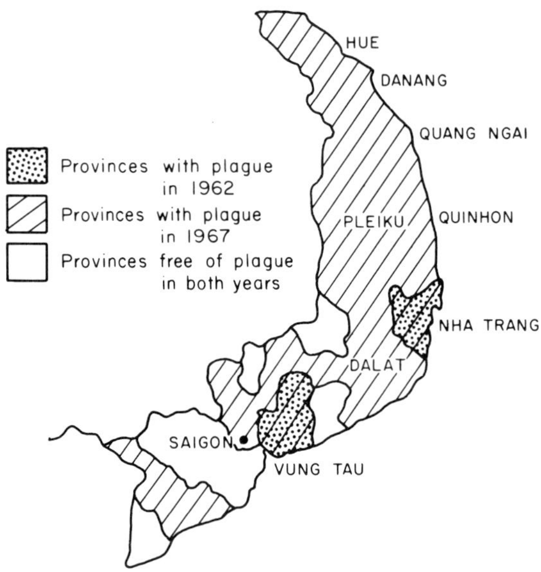

Figure 3.3. The spread of human plague infection in Vietnam after 1962 from limited foci of southern and eastern areas to the northern and western areas of the country.

> have been reported as positive in 7.5% of confirmed bubonic plague patients and in 12.3% of asymptomatic contacts. The epidemiological importance of these findings is not yet clear and the facts need verification. Several outbreaks of plague pneumonia were seen from 1964 onwards, a small outbreak in Long Khan and a mixed bubonic–pneumonic epidemic in Binh-Dinh province in the central highland village of An Khe . . . .
>
> It is believed that the transportation of grains and rice between village and town played a major role in the spread of plague to cities. However, unusual living conditions created by war have brought into close and intimate contact humans and an extremely abundant rodent population. (pp. 493–497)

A sharp decline in the number of reported cases in Vietnam occurred in 1972, as shown in Table 3.1. Whether vaccination of the people with a locally produced vaccine (EV strain, which was given to an estimated 25,000,000 people, or about 43% of the people in infected areas) played a role in the decline of cases is uncertain. The observed decline of cases could have been the result of a normal biological cycle of plague in the rodent populations, as has been observed at 5-year intervals in other countries.

Although plague became widespread in Vietnam after 1965, a focal geographic pattern was maintained at most times. For instance, during the period 1972–1975, nearly all the cases of plague referred to the Cho-Quan Hospital in Saigon originated from a focus in the town of Cu Chi, located about 30 miles from Saigon in Hau Nghia Province.

3.1.3.2. Factors Influencing the Spread of Plague in Vietnam

At the Symposium on plague in Saigon in 1970, Dr. Nguyen Dang Que presented the following three factors responsible for the spread of plague:

1. Security problem. North Vietnamese troops had been infiltrating and covertly operated within the territory of the Republic of Vietnam. This was the cause of the lack of security in several places to which health teams could not go to work.
2. Transportation network. Vehicles carried goods from remote villages to cities, junks and boats transported goods between coastal cities, planes shared in the transportation of passengers, and highways were built. Thus, plague spread from provinces, which were considered as foci, to neighboring provinces along the ways of communication and highways.
3. Refugees. An estimated 6,000,000 people in Vietnam were forced to move from their farmland to the cities. Concomitant with the increase of the population in provincial capitals and cities, houses

popped up rapidly and in a disorderly fashion. Minimum sanitary requirements were not met. Many large families were packed into small housing units where garbage was thrown pell-mell and not disposed of. These were favorable conditions for rats to feed and breed.

The authorities could not make adequate manpower available for the destruction of rats and for the appropriate disposal of garbage. Given the above conditions, the problem of control of plague was insoluble.

The widespread use of chemical sprays for defoliation during the Vietnam war could be another factor in the spread of plague. Although this factor was not carefully evaluated, it is clear that the natural habitats and food supplies of field rodents were drastically altered by the defoliants. This could have produced changes in rodent populations that led to a resurgence of plague infection in the remaining rodent populations.

3.1.3.3. Reservoirs and Vectors

The major rodent reservoirs of plague in Vietnam were *R. norvegicus, R. exulans,* and the house shrew *Suncus murinus*. These species were trapped in urban areas of Vietnam. Tissues of about 0.4% of all three were bacteriologically positive for *Y. pestis*. Likewise, fleas obtained from 0.2–0.3% of these rodents were positive for *Y. pestis*. In adjacent foothills surrounding the city of Nha Trang, the burrowing feral rodent *Bandicota indica* (bandicoot) was also trapped. Tissues from 2 of 18 bandicoots and one flea were positive for *Y. pestis,* suggesting the possible interchange of infected fleas from urban and sylvatic rodents.[8]

Fleas obtained from these rodents were predominantly the oriental rat flea *Xenopsylla cheopis*. A few *Xenopsylla astia* were also obtained.

3.1.3.4. Seasonal Trends

Plague in Vietnam exhibited a striking seasonality that was nearly the same throughout the country. The peak incidence occurred in March and April with far fewer cases in all other months. This time coincided with the warm–dry time of year. Before this time it was cool and rainy, and after this time it became very hot. During the peak months of March and April, the flea index of *R. norvegicus* in Saigon increased from one or less to about three fleas per rat. In Nha Trang during April of 1966 these rats exhibited a flea index of more than eight fleas per rat![9–10]

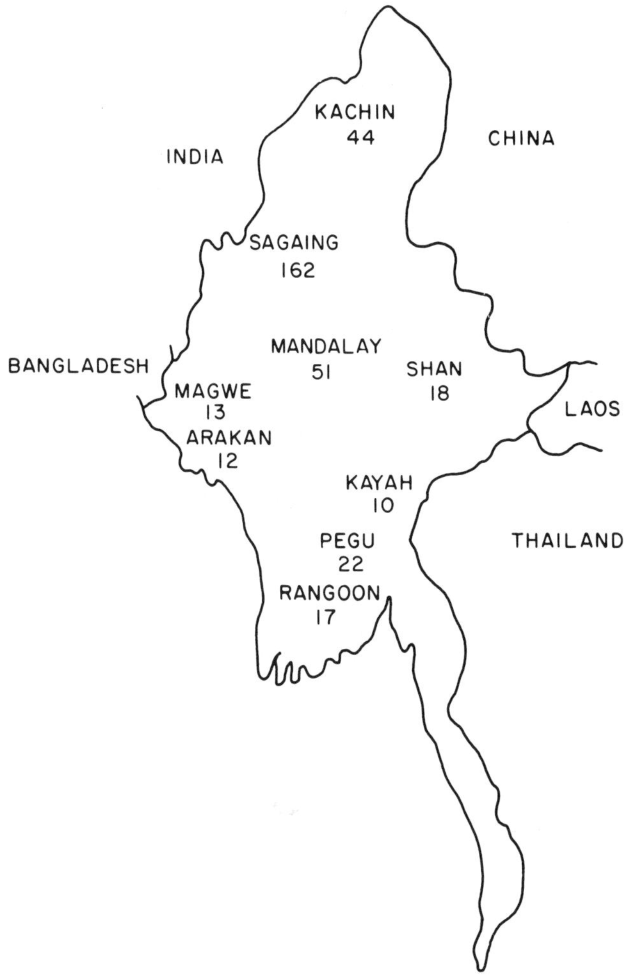
KACHIN
44
CHINA
INDIA
SAGAING
162
MANDALAY
51
BANGLADESH
SHAN
18
MAGWE
13
LAOS
ARAKAN
12
KAYAH
10
PEGU
22
THAILAND
RANGOON
17

Figure 3.4. The distribution of confirmed human plague cases in Burma in the first half of 1977. The numbers refer to the numbers of human cases. This information was provided by Dr. K. Arnold and Dr. Seinyi (personal communication).

3.1.4. Plague in Burma

The large numbers of cases of human plague reported from Burma in recent years, as high as 700 cases in 1974, indicates that this country has been second only to Vietnam in the incidence of plague. Like Vietnam, plague was officially recorded in Burma in 1898, when it was reportedly imported from India. Plague has been continuously endemic and sporadically epidemic in Burma ever since. According to Velimirovic,[6] there were more than 165,400 recorded deaths from plague between 1905 and 1940. All areas of the country have been infected, but since 1946 the disease has occurred predominantly in northern and central Burma.

In the first half of 1977 confirmed cases of human plague have been documented in several areas of Burma, as shown in Figure 3.4. The largest number of cases occurred in the northern division of Sagaing. Of the 355 confirmed cases in Burma in 1977, deaths were recorded in 22 persons, or 6%. An outbreak in Hlegu in 1977 near Rangoon, affected 14 people, causing two deaths.[11] A ratfall (die-off) in the market preceded the outbreak. Most cases were male children.

Both field rodents and domestic rodents are believed to be involved in plague epizootics in Burma. A survey in 1948 showed positive cultures from *R. rattus* and *Bandicota bengalensis*. In Ragoon there is a Rodent Control Demonstration Unit operated by the World Health Organization which has reported plague infection in both rodents and human.[12,13] The most numerous rodents in Rangoon were *R. rattus, R. exulans, R. norvegicus, B. bengalensis,* and *S. murinus*. The flea vectors were predominantly *X. astia* and *X. cheopis*. The flea indices for these host species exceeded one flea per rodent in nearly all determinations.

3.1.5. Plague in Brazil

3.1.5.1. History

Plague was introduced into Brazil by ships during the epidemic originating in China in the 1890s. The disease occurred in the coastal seaport cities including Rio de Janeiro, but was brought under control, in part, by public health programs that used rat control. Subsequently foci of the disease became established in mostly rural areas of northeastern Brazil, predominantly in the states of Bahia, Pernambuco, and Ceara.

3.1.5.2. Occurrence and Distribution

The epidemiology of plague in Brazil was studied well by Machiavello in 1939–1940[14] and more recently by Almedia *et al.*[15] During the last decade, Brazil has reported more human plague than other countries in the

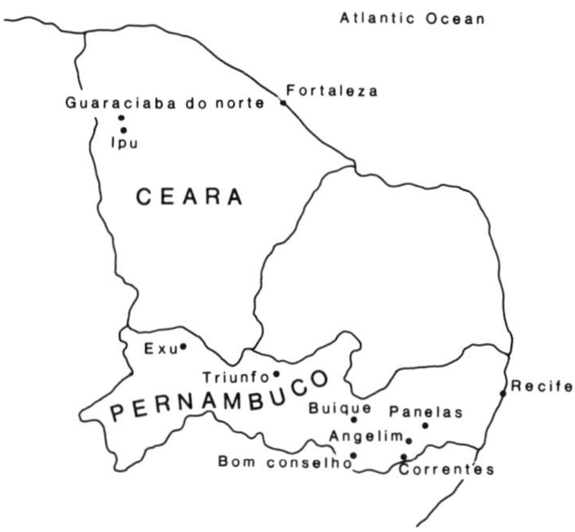

Figure 3.5. Foci of plague infection in the states of Pernambuco and Ceara in northeastern Brazil. The coastal cities of Fortaleza and Recife are plague-free and are shown for the purpose of orientation only.

western hemisphere and according to the data for the entire world in Table 3.1, ranks third in the occurrence of plague, behind only Vietnam and Burma.

Cycles of plague at an occurrence of every 5–10 years have been noted in Brazil. The variation of reported human plague (as shown in Table 3.1) suggests that a high point of activity occurred in 1975, when 496 cases were

TABLE 3.2
Human Plague in Ceara State of Brazil: Patients with Fever and Bubo Who Had Elevated Convalescent Passive Hemagglutination (PHA) Titers against Fraction I of *Y. pestis*

Date of illness	Date of serum collection	Reciprocal of PHA titer	Age	Sex
Dec. 77	May 78	256[a]	65	F
Jan. 78	May 78	64	18	F
Jan. 78	May 78	≥128	56	M
Feb. 78	May 78	≥128	44	F
Feb. 78	Jun. 78	128	38	M
Feb. 78	Jun. 78	128	26	M
Apr. 78	Jun. 78	64	2	M
Apr. 78	May 78	64	2	F
Apr. 78	Jun. 78	128	18	M
May 78	Jun. 78	16	11	M
May 78	Jun. 78	32	6	M

[a] This patient had a positive blood culture for *Y. pestis* during the acute illness.

confirmed, whereas there was a paucity of cases in the following years. Nevertheless, human plague was occurring in Ceara State at the end of the decade, as a retrospective serological study showed in 1978 (Table 3.2).

The geographic distribution of known plague foci in the states of Pernambuco and Ceara during the decade 1970–1979 is shown in Figure 3.5. These are rural areas with hills and farmlands. The majority of human cases in the latter years of decade 1970–1979 occurred on the Ibiapaba plateau of Ceara State, including the town of Ipu and Guaraciaba do Norte, at an altitude of about 1000 m.[(16)]

3.1.5.3. Reservoirs and Vectors

Although Macchivello[(14)] found *R. rattus* to be the most important reservoir for plague in rural Brazil, Almeida and his co-workers found that *Zygodontomys pixuna,* a burrowing field rodent, carried plague more often and was involved in die-offs during epizootics. *Zygodontomys pixuna* was shown to be more susceptible to experimental plague than were rats, suggesting that these field rodents spread plague during epizootics but that other more resistant animals must be the major enzootic reservoir.[(16)] Contact between the field rodents and domestic rats is believed to be responsible for the transmission of plague to man. Flea vectors have been examined in Brazil by pooling fleas from captured wild rodents in northeast Brazil, and such flea pools have been culture-positive for *Y. pestis.* The most common fleas are *X. cheopis* and *X. brasiliensis.*

3.1.5.4. Seasonal Variation

Although some cases of human plague in Brazil during 1970–1979 occurred during all months of the year, the majority of the cases occurred in October–December. This is the warm–dry season which corresponds also to the season when farmers are harvesting their crops of sugarcane and corn. At this time of year, people are, therefore, more frequently in contact with field rodents.

3.1.5.5. Host Factors

In northeast Brazil during the latter years of the last decade, plague cases showed a preponderance of males that was most evident in the children between the ages of 5 and 15 years. In the adults, there was a more even sex distribution.[15] Most cases occurred in farmers and their families, and most of them were derived from the Indian or Negro races. This racial distribution reflects the makeup of the population of poor farmers in this region. It suggests that exposure to plague may be the explanation for the occurrence of plague infection in these peoples, rather than any racial predisposition.

3.1.6. Plague in the United States

3.1.6.1. History

Plague arrived in the United States in 1900 by ship from China to San Francisco.[2] The first recorded case was in a Chinese worker who lived in Chinatown, and by 1902 about 100 more cases had occurred. By 1905 121 people were known to have been infected and 118 of them had died. Rat-proofing of houses was begun and the outbreak was curtailed. There were, however, smaller epidemics in California in 1907, 1919, and 1924. During this time the infection spread to sylvatic rodents, such as prairie dogs and ground squirrels, of California and adjacent states as far as Kansas. All of the human plague in the United States after 1925 (except for rare laboratory accidents and imported cases) has occurred in nonurban sylvatic foci.

3.1.6.2. Occurrence and Distribution

The numbers of human cases in the United States by decade from 1900 to 1979 are shown in Table 3.3. After the urban outbreaks in California up

TABLE 3.3
Numbers of Cases of Human Plague in the United States from 1900 to 1979

Decade	Cases
1900–1909	332
1910–1919	69
1920–1929	99
1930–1939	10
1940–1949	10
1950–1959	10
1960–1969	28
1970–1979	105

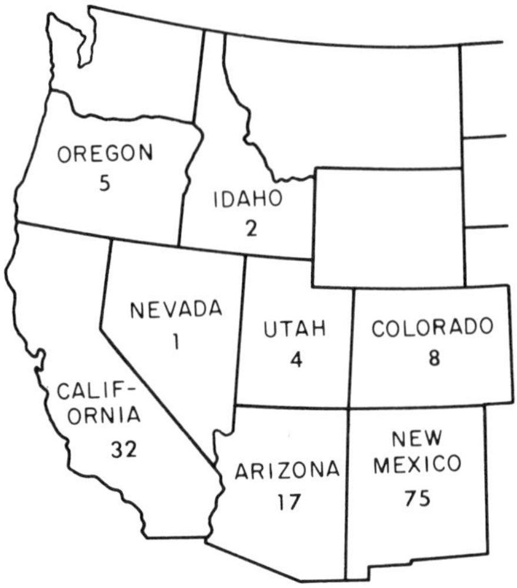
OREGON
5
IDAHO
2
NEVADA
1
UTAH
4
COLORADO
8
CALIF-
ORNIA
32
ARIZONA
17
NEW
MEXICO
75

Figure 3.6. Confirmed human cases of plague reported by state in the United States between 1925 and 1977.

to 1924, there were very few cases (10 per decade) until the 1960s and 1970s when there was a resurgence.[17–19] In recent years, as shown in Table 3.1, there have been 16–18 cases a year. The same trend has persisted since these years. In 1980, there were 18 reported cases; in 1981, 13 cases; and in 1982, 19 cases.

The geographic distribution of the cases by state after 1925 is shown in Figure 3.6. New Mexico showed more cases than any other state. Before 1970, however, California had contributed the majority of the cases. Only in this last decade has New Mexico emerged as the leading state for human plague when it has accounted for about 50% of all cases in the United States.

3.1.6.3. Reservoirs and Vectors

Plague-infected animals were found in association with 32 human cases between 1900 and 1966.[17,18,20] Ground squirrels were near the houses of 12 persons, ground squirrels were in the same county as 13 others, wood rats and grasshopper mice were near the homes of two cases each, and in one case each, a chipmunk, rabbit, marmot, or pack rat was near the home. Infected fleas were found near the homes of six persons.

Kartman reviewed the information on animal reservoirs in 1970.[18] The colonizing rodents, the ground squirrel and the prairie dog, were most commonly observed and were associated with human cases. However, the more important reservoir of *Y. pestis* in nature appeared to be the meadow vole *Microtus californicus,* which was relatively resistant to infection and carried large numbers of fleas.

Between 1970 and 1979 several isolations of *Y. pestis* from animals and fleas were made during the epidemiological investigations of human cases.[20–25] Dead animals, with bacteria in their tissues, that were found nearby or that patients had handled have included a bobcat, a coyote, a rabbit, a rock squirrel, ground squirrels, tree squirrels, a cat, a pack rat, and wood rats. Culture-positive fleas were discovered on a pack rat, wood rats, field mice, rabbits, and a rock squirrel, and in an abandoned rodent burrow. The fleas that are the important vectors from the animal reservoirs to man in the United States are *Diamanus montanus* and *Hoplopsyllus anomalus*.[25a]

Although rabbits are associated classically with tularemia rather than plague, von Reyn *et al.* reported eight patients with plague who had contact with infected rabbits.[22] The mode of acquisition of the infection by hand contact resulted in a different pattern of epidemiologic and clinical features (see Table 3.4).

TABLE 3.4
Features of Rabbit-Associated Plague Cases Compared to Other Plague Cases in the United States 1950–1974[a]

	Rabbit-associated cases (8 patients)	All other plague cases (58 patients)
Ages of patients	All >20 years	Most <20 years
Male : female ratio	7 : 1	1.4 : 1
Seasonal peak	Winter	Summer
Exposure	Tissue contact with rabbit	Usually unknown or rodent contact or flea bite
Site of bubo	Axillary or epitrochlear	Usually femoral or inguinal
Case–fatality rate	50%	17%

[a] Adapted from von Reyn *et al.*[22] with permission of publisher.

3.1.6.4. Seasonal Distribution

Between 1950 and 1975, 84% of patients who were associated with wild animals and their fleas became ill between May and September. This is the warm time of year when people are outdoors more than at other times and it is also the time of year when epizootics have occurred in the animal populations. On the other hand, the seasonal distribution of plague associated with handling or skinning dead animals has a less distinct pattern. Several cases had their onset in the winter, during the hunting seasons for rabbits and carnivores.

3.1.6.5. Risk Factors for Human Plague

All ages and both sexes of humans are highly susceptible to plague infection following sufficient exposure. The age distribution of plague shows that children are particularly susceptible: 65% of cases between 1925 and 1975 were less than 20 years old. The youngest case was 7 days old. In the United States, males have predominated over females by a ratio of about 2 : 1. This sex predilection may be only differential exposure because it was striking in adults, whereas children showed a more nearly equal sex distribution. Actually, during the decade of the 1970s, slightly more than half of the cases in the United States were females, thus ending the earlier male preponderance.[26]

Human contact with rodent reservoirs and their fleas has been studied as a logical risk factor in developing infection. Mann and co-workers looked for evidence of animal contacts in 16 patients with plague in New Mexico by a retrospective case–control method.[27] Only two patients reported direct skin contact with animal tissues. In the others, there was no evidence that seeing rodents around the home or having non-rodent-proof homes played any role in infection. Patients did, however, live in places that provided opportunities for rodent harborage and food more frequently than did the controls. Furthermore, the patients less often took measures to control fleas on their domestic pets. Whether these risk factors of providing rodents with food and harborage and of not controlling fleas on pets were merely associated with human plague infection or were directly contributory to human infection could not be determined in this study. From their results, Mann *et al.* concluded that plague infection probably resulted from infected rodents entering the habitat of man rather than from man entering the sylvatic habits of the animals. These findings are also consistent with the suggestion of von Reyn *et al.*[24] that domestic dogs and cats may acquire infected fleas from wild rodents and thus transmit the infection to man. Although the majority of cases occurred in white persons, about a fourth of the cases have been in American Indians. Thus, the incidence of plague in the Indian population is much greater than in whites. This relatively high incidence of plague in Indians can be attributed to the rural location and living conditions of these people in the southwestern states. Kartman has reported an outbreak in 1965, involving six Indians in New Mexico, that was associated with infected prairie dogs and their fleas.[18]

The case–fatality rate of human plague in the United States during 1970–1979 was 15/105 (14%). Fatal infection was more common in patients who were over 60 years old (57%). Death rates by sex and race did not show notable differences.[26]

3.1.7. Plague in Indonesia

Although there were only ten human cases reported from Indonesia during the decade of the 1970s (Table 3.1), Indonesia is an important region for plague because of the epidemic of 1968 that produced 102 confirmed human cases. All of these cases were clustered in mountain villages of the Boyolali Regency of central Java. Epidemiological studies by Williams and his co-workers[28] have revealed many interesting facets of this focus of infection.

Plague was introduced into Java in 1910 and spread rapidly to produce large epidemics in 1915 and 1923. Between 1911 and 1939 there were recorded 217,550 cases of human plague, making Indonesia one of the leading Asian countries for the occurrence of this infection during this century.

There were no reported human cases in Indonesia, however, from 1961 to 1967. Then the disease reappeared in mountainous villages in the volcanic range of Boyolali Regency of central Java. The infected people lived at altitudes of greater than 1000 m. They were farmers in an area of intensive agriculture and dense population. No medical facilities were available during the epidemic, and the case–fatality rate was 35% in the reported plague cases. The majority of cases occurred during January and February.

Studies of rodent reservoirs revealed that plague occurred predominantly in rats of two species: *R. rattus* and *R. exulans* carried plague at altitudes above 1000 m, whereas only *R. rattus* was found to harbor infection at lower altitudes. The fleas *X. cheopis* and *Stivalius cognatus* that were obtained from rodents were shown to be infected. Rodent surveys from 1972 to 1974 showed that plague infection remained enzootic, but there have been no human cases reported since 1971 in Indonesia. It is likely, however, that this focus of plague infection may erupt again to cause human cases in the future. The interepidemic persistence of plague has been an elusive subject for investigators, but the infection certainly does persist in geographic areas that have no apparent epidemic activity for many years. Plague bacilli can survive for long periods in the soil, and burrowing rodents may contract infection either by eating other dead rodents or through mucous membrane contact with contaminated soil.[29]

3.1.8. Ecology of Plague

Although man's primary reason for studying plague is that it is a serious disease of man, the understanding of the epidemiology of plague and of the implications for disease control requires study of the natural animal reservoirs and flea vectors that transmit the infection among the reservoir hosts. With only rare exceptions, man is an accidental host and plays no role in the maintenance or propagation of plague in nature. Accordingly, most of the work on the epidemiology of plague has been conducted in the field to define animal hosts, flea vectors, and patterns of transmission in the natural habitats of many countries. Reviews of this subject after Pollitzer's monograph in 1954 have been written by Baltazard, Bahmanyar, and Kartman *et al.*[5,18,30] This subject is so complex that Garnham stated in 1949, "The ecology of wild rodent plague is most complex; to unravel it is like following the different voices in a Bach fugue, except that in plague the basic design is unknown."[31]

3.1.8.1. Animal Reservoirs

In the entire history of urban human plague, the domestic black rat *R. rattus* has probably been the most important host. It climbs well, inhabits ships as well as houses, and is a good host for the efficient plague flea vector *X. cheopis*. Plague in other than the urban setting, however, has taken on many complex variations. The classic theory of plague reservoirs requires one or more relatively resistant small mammal species, which serve as the enzootic reservoir species, and one or more relatively susceptible species, which serve as the epizootic hosts and may be involved in the so-called rat die-offs or ratfalls. In urban plague the same species of rats can be both the enzootic and epizootic species, whereas in rural or sylvatic plague, there are usually two or more separate species. For example, in India Baltazard and Bahmanyar found that the field gerbil *Tatera indica* was resistant to plague and served as the enzootic reservoir. The domestic rats were "liaison rodents," carrying plague from gerbils to man.[(5)] In Java, the resistant field species was *R. exulans* and, again, the domestic rats were merely liaisons to man.[(32)] In the sylvatic plague that occurs in the United States, the ecology of plague does not neatly fit this pattern. Although the colonizing rodents, ground squirrels, and prairie dogs have frequently brought plague to man, the resistant enzootic species has been difficult to define. Kartman *et al.* suggested that the meadow vole was responsible for enzooticity in California.[(30)] More recently in New Mexico and Arizona, the carnivorous coyotes and bobcats, as well as rabbits, were shown to be infected with plague, but the modes of transmission among these animals remain to be delineated.

In Vietnam the brown street rat *R. norvegicus* was an important plague reservoir, in addition to *R. rattus*. The house shrew *S. murinus* also carried plague and appeared to be an important host for carrying infection to man.[(33,34)]

In Africa, the wild rodent complex *Mastomys natalensis* has been demonstrated to be an important reservoir for the maintenance of both plague and the virus of Lassa fever by Green and co-workers.[(35)] Isaacson *et al.*[(36)] in South Africa examined the susceptibility of *Mastomys* to experimental plague infection and found that *M. natalensis* was relatively resistant to fatal infection, as shown by a 50% death rate after a dose of 1.9×10^5 bacteria given subcutaneously. By contrast, another species called *Mastomys coucha,* which differs from other species by having diploid chromosomes of numbers 32 and 36, was susceptible to death when inoculated with only 1.9×10^2 bacteria. This suggests that genetically determined differences among species of rodents could allow the same genus to provide a relatively resistant enzootic reservoir and a more susceptible epizootic reservoir for plague infection.

Some of the fluctuations in plague occurrence have been related to changing populations of the rodent reservoirs. In Indian cities, Seal described replacement of *R. rattus* by *B. bengalensis* at the same time that human plague diminished.[(37)] Although both rodents were good hosts for *Y. pestis, R. rattus* was more heavily parasitized with the efficient flea vector *X. cheopis* than were the bandicoot rats. The virtual elimination of plague infection from India after 1950 was an astonishing event and could have other explanations. One possibility is that insecticide spraying to control mosquitoes as vectors of malaria also had a controlling effect on the fleas that transmitted plague.

In Japan, the last recorded case of human plague occurred in 1926 and the last case of rodent plague in 1930. A serological survey of rats by Suzuki and Hotta[38] from 1971 to 1977 revealed that four *R. norvegicus* rodents showed positive results. However, no isolations of *Y. pestis* could be made, and these results suggest that the antiplague antibody tests using Fraction I antigen are not entirely specific for plague.

3.1.8.2. Flea Vectors

The Commission for the Investigation of Plague in India established that the oriental rat flea *X. cheopis* was the most important vector of plague transmission. The reason that this was an efficient vector was shown by Bacot and Martin in 1914.[39] They showed that several days after ingesting infected rat blood the proventriculus of these fleas became obstructed by a solid mass of plague bacteria. Thus, these fleas were "blocked," so that subsequent blood feedings could not pass into the stomach. Nevertheless, the blocked fleas tried to feed and regurgitated blood, which was contaminated by their own bacteria in the obstructed proventriculus, back into the wound. Not satisfying their thirst, they made repeated bites. Through this blocking mechanism *X. cheopis* was a more efficient vector than another rat flea *Ceratophyllus fasciatus*. Blocked fleas could live for 23 days at 27°C with high humidity, but died rapidly from dessication at higher temperatures or in dryer conditions. This climatic effect on blocked fleas could explain why plague epidemics are terminated by very hot and dry weather, and Kartman showed that fleas at 23.5°C were better vectors than at 29.5°C with regard to duration of their infection, development of blocking, longevity after blocking, and likelihood of transmitting the infection.[40] This effect of temperature on the blocking of infected fleas has been related further by Cavanaugh to activation of enzymes of both the plague bacillus and the flea stomach.[41] The coagulase of *Y. pestis,* which contributes to the clotting of blood in the flea, was active at 25°C but not at 37°C, whereas a fibrinolytic factor of *Y. pestis,* which dissolves blood clots, was active at 37°C but not at 25°C. A trypsinlike enzyme of the flea stomach was also more active at 37°C and may contribute to the lysis of clots at the higher temperatures. Thus, the coagulation of ingested blood, which is believed to be a necessary early event in the process of blocking of the alimentary tract of the flea, appears to be enzymatically abrogated at higher temperatures (above 25°C) and may play a role in the seasonal attributes of plague epidemics.

Although the blocking of fleas by *Y. pestis* appears to be important in nature, other means of flea transmission may occur. These include penetration of the infected flea feces into abraded skin and the mechanical transmission through biting with infected flea mouth parts. Kartman *et al.* showed that for sylvatic plague near San Francisco the flea *Hystrichopsylla linsdalei* transmitted infection by the blocking mechanism, but that another flea *Malaraeus telchinum* probably transmitted infection by mechanical biting.[30]

Another part of the complex ecology of plague is the relationship of the potential flea vectors to their mammalian hosts. Generally, the flea species that are narrowly adapted to a particular host are so poorly adapted to man that they have only transient existences on man, but this can, of course, be long enough for a few bites and the transmission of plague. The human flea *Pulex irritans* is not an efficient plague vector and rarely, if ever, has transmitted plague from man to man. Table 3.5 shows some of the important flea vectors of the world.

The proliferation of fleas on rodents is believed to be crucial for the propagation of plague epidemics. Much has been made of the flea index (the average number of fleas per rodent). When the flea index is high, that is, exceeding one, the chances for an epizootic among rodents is greater. The multiplication of fleas on rodents is highly seasonal, being greatest in the warm and dry times when epidemics are most likely to occur. In Vietnam,

TABLE 3.5
Some Important Flea Vectors for Transmission of Plague[a]

Species	Distribution	Hosts
Xenopsylla cheopis	Worldwide, especially in tropics	Rats
Xenopsylla brasiliensis	South America, Africa, India	Rats
Xenopsylla astia	Southeast Asia	Rats
Xenopsylla vexabilis	Pacific islands	Rats
Pulex irritans[b]	Worldwide	Wide range, including man
Nosopsyllus fasciatus	Worldwide	Rats
Malaraeus telchinum	United States	Sylvatic rodents
Diamanus montanus	United States	Sylvatic rodents
Hoplopsyllus anomalus	United States	Sylvatic rodents
Stivalius cognatus	Indonesia	Rats
Polygenis species	Brazil	Field rodents

[a] Adapted from Bahmanyar and Cavanaugh.[3]
[b] Postulated as a vector by Blanc and Baltazard[47] and Ell.[48] See Section 3.1.8.4.

the rainy season curtailed sharply the transmission of plague and concomitantly reduced flea indices.[42]

Although rodent fleas are specific for their host species and, thus, are rarely exchanged, the intermingling of different rodent species and their fleas has been observed in the field and might explain the migration of plague from an urban focus to a sylvatic focus, and vice versa. The dangers of transferring plague from wild rodents back to domestic rodents (and next to man!) have been long recognized. The wild rodent flea *M. telchinum* was found on the urban rat *R. norvegicus* in San Francisco in 1938.[30] Also in California, Meyer and his colleagues found that rats harbored two species of fleas that were native to ground squirrels, suggesting that rodents of entirely different habitats exchanged their fleas. Furthermore, rodent fleas have been found on dogs. Fleas of domestic dogs and cats have been implicated in the transmission of plague to man in the United States,[24] but infection of these fleas with *Y. pestis* has only rarely been identified.

3.1.8.3. Oral Transmission

Transmission of plague by ingestion was recognized by Yersin and Kitasato in their original descriptions of the plague bacillus in 1894 (see Chapter 2). They fed pieces of liver and spleen of infected animals to other rats or mice, which then developed fatal infections. Rust *et al.* found that dogs and cats were also susceptible to experimental infection by the oral route.[43] These experimental results suggest that *Y. pestis* can cross the gastrointestinal mucosa to cause infection and that transmission in nature could occur without flea vectors by carnivores ingesting infected tissues. Carnivores have, indeed, been infected naturally and linked to human infections in the United States,[25] but this mode of transmission is believed to be tangential to the major enzootic reservoirs of noncarnivorous rodents. Other possible modes of transmission include a fecal–oral route, but feces and intestinal contents of orally infected animals have not yielded positive cultures for *Y. pestis*.[43a] Burrowing rodents might otherwise have nasal or oral mucous membrane contact with infected soil of their burrows, in which *Y. pestis* has been shown to survive for periods of up to a year following an epizootic.[4,44,45]

3.1.8.4. Human-to-Human Transmission

Although the most common route of human infection is from infected rodent fleas, outbreaks of plague pneumonia spread by infected airborne droplets or aerosols have occurred. Fortunately, this mode of man-to-man transmission is rare and seems to be short-lived, because in part, plague pneumonia is so rapidly fatal that the victims have little time to spread their infection to others. The potential of a human reservoir of respiratory plague infection was suggested by Marshall and co-workers in Vietnam, who demonstrated the pharyngeal carrier state.[46] They showed that 16 of 212 patients with bubonic plague had positive throat cultures for *Y. pestis,* as did 15 of 114 healthy contacts of patients. The pharyngeal carrier state persisted for as long as 21 days. None of these pharyngeal carriers developed pneumonic plague, and there was no evidence that they were contagious. However, these studies point out the alarming possibility of a silent human reservoir from which pneumonic plague epidemics could erupt.

Another form of interhuman plague transmission, directly via fleas, was studied in the Kurdish peoples by Blanc and Baltazard. They presented evidence that the human flea *P. irritans* may transmit the disease from man to man.[47] This mode of transmission must be rare and must require extremely unhygienic and crowded living conditions. Nevertheless, this postulated means of transmission deserves some attention as a possible explanation for ancient epidemics that occurred under conditions that may have favored the exchange of human fleas more than is possible today. In fact, this sort of historical presentation has been advanced recently by Ell for the medieval plague epidemics.[48] According to this argument, human flea transmission, rather than either rat flea or respiratory droplet transmission, should be associated with interpersonal spread of the bubonic presentation, seasonal occurrence in times other than the summer or winter, large numbers of cases per household, and the absence of rat mortality. Medieval European texts actually do support this thesis, but the absence of scientific accuracy in these nonmedical texts does not allow us to exclude that the more accepted modes of modern times (i.e., rat flea and respiratory droplet transmissions) might have occurred also during medieval times.

3.1.8.5. Human Host Factors in Plague Transmission

Human plague infection occurs predominantly in groups of people living under adverse conditions of poverty, crowding, malnutrition, and other diseases. Although increased exposure of these groups of people to rat fleas may explain in large part their susceptibility to plague infection, it must also be considered that decreased host defenses against infection play a role in these groups. Malnutrition is known to depress immune reactions, and other infections, such as malaria and tuberculosis, may also exert immunosuppressive effects on the host defenses, rendering such people more susceptible to plague infection.

3.1.9. Mortality from Plague

A hallmark of human plague infection is a high case–fatality rate. Yersin's original description of *Y. pestis* in Hong Kong in 1894 mentions a 95% case–fatality rate for hospitalized cases (see Chapter 2). Although this rate is much higher than that of all human plague infection, which includes a spectrum of mild disease and even asymptomatic infection, patients with plague disease have a high risk of dying. Antibiotics have reduced the risk of death when administered early in the course of the disease.

Accurate data on mortality rates are not available because population denominators are often not known and confirmation of suspected cases of plague is often difficult. In the first half of this century, India was the dominant country for incidence of and fatality from plague. An estimated 10,000,000 human deaths from plague occurred in India, and as late as 1953, 78% of the world's cases were reported from India. Since 1967, there have been no recorded cases in India, representing a remarkable and unknown feature of the biological cycles that govern plague epidemiology (for possible explanations, see the discussion of animal reservoirs in Section 3.1.8.1). A summary of case–fatality rates for plague, as reported by the World Health Organization, was presented by Akiev.[48a] In the period 1966–1978, there were 2067 deaths from plague, or a case–fatality rate of 5.4%. This is almost certainly an underestimate of the true case–fatality rate because rates are higher in individual countries that have antibiotics available for early use in the disease. In countries with antibiotic usage, antibiotics are often not used early enough to prevent death, and these countries probably report deaths more accurately than do countries that have less antibiotic usage. Between 1966 and 1978 in Burma, the case–fatality rate was 11%. In Indonesia, the case–fatality rate was 42% and in Nepal 78%. In the Americas, it was 14%, whereas for the continent of Africa it was 22%. Within Africa, Madagascar reported a 34% case–fatality rate and Zaire reported 20%. This considerable variation in the recorded mortality from plague indicates that in the best situations of health care facilities, fatalities will occur in the range of 5–15% of all cases. The rapidly progressive nature in *Y. pestis* infection in man means that antibiotic therapy may not be able to reduce case–fatality rates further than this level.

3.2. *YERSINIA ENTEROCOLITICA* INFECTION

Our understanding of the epidemiology of this infection is in its infancy when compared to that of plague because only recently has it been possible to identify and study the disease in populations. From the first human case described in 1939 by Schleifstein and Coleman[48b] until 1975, there were only 84 cases reported in the United States and about 6000 cases in the world literature.[49] The actual incidence of this infection is unknown because it is not a reportable disease. Furthermore, it is underdiagnosed on account of its protean clinial manifestations and the failure of physicians and laboratories to pursue a bacteriological diagnosis in an appropriate setting. From what is known at the present time, it is clear that the epidemiology of *Y. enterocolitica* differs sharply from that of plague by having both human and animal reservoirs (principally, the pig), by being excreted in feces and transmitted by ingestion, and by not having any known invertebate vectors involved in its transmission. Furthermore, plague occurs predominantly in tropical and developing countries, whereas nonplague yersinioses are more prevalent in developed countries where meat products, especially pork, are handled and stored before being ingested.

3.2.1. Geographic Distribution

Yersinia enterocolitica appears to have a worldwide distribution. The majority of the reported cases have originated from Europe, especially Sweden, Belgium, and France, where diagnostic interest and the use of methodology is particularly high. For example, in Belgium there were 1781 culture-proven cases between 1963 and 1975, as reported by Vandepitte and Wauters,[50] and in France there were only 168 culture-proven cases from 1967–1977, as reported by Alonso *et al.*[51] Many cases have also been reported from Canada, Finland, Denmark, South Africa, the United States, and Japan. In the United States, *Y. enterocolitica* isolations from human cases have been documented from many regions of that country. The states with at least five proven cases during the last decade include New York, Wisconsin, Washington, California, North Carolina, Pennsylvania, Tennessee, Arkansas, and Mississippi.

In recent years, cases of *Y. enterocolitica* infection have been reported from tropical countries of Africa, Asia and South America, but these infections do not appear to have a high incidence in tropical countries. Cases of *Y. enterocolitica* infection have been reported from Zaire by Makulu *et al.*,[52] from Nigeria by Agbonlahor *et al.*[53] and Anjorin *et al.*,[54] and from Bangladesh (T. Butler, unpublished observations). The first known case from Brazil occurred in 1976, as reported by Pizsolitto *et al.*[55]

Estimates of the incidence of yersiniosis have been made in Denmark and Finland by carrying out serological surveys. Agner *et al.*[56] tested sera from adults in Denmark from 1967 to 1978 and found that the prevalence of elevated antibody titers against *Y. enterocolitica* O:3 had increased from 1% in 1967 to 7.7% in 1978. The prevalence was higher in females than males, and the titers were highest in the autumn, which is the same time of year that pigs are most frequently infected. In Finland, Leino[57] showed that elevated agglutinin titers against *Y. enterocolitica* O:3 or O:9 or against *Y. pseudotuberculosis* IA occurred in 6.1% of all sera tested, with a range from 3.2 to 8.5% in each year from 1971 to 1978. Although these serological studies may not be specific for yersiniosis and do not give an accurate incidence of infection, they suggest that yersiniosis is common and widespread among the people of northern Europe.

3.2.2. Serotypes and Biotypes

There are 34 O serotypes of *Y. enterocolitica,* but only a few of these serotypes have been isolated from human sources. In Europe, the predominant human serotypes are O:3 and O:9, in Canada and Japan O:3; whereas in the United States, the majority of reported infections have been caused by serotype O:8, with the exception that Bissett [57a] found serotype O:5,27 to be the most common one in California. In Canada, serotypes O:5,27 and O:6,30 are occasionally isolated from humans. In South Africa, serotypes O:5 and O:6 have been isolated from human cases[58] and in Norway these serotypes as well as O:4, O:7,8, and O:13,7 were isolated from feces of healthy persons,[59] but the pathogenic role of *Y. enterocolitica* strains belonging to serotypes other than O:3, O:8, and O:9 remains unclear.

There are five biotypes of *Y. enterocolitica* which are based on biochemical reactions that affect utilization of indole, xylose, and trehalose and

TABLE 3.6
Predominant Serotypes and Biotypes of *Yersinia enterocolitica* Found in Human Cases in Different Countries

Country	O serotypes	Biotypes
Bangladesh	7,8	
Belgium	3; 9; 6; 5	
Brazil	3	4
Canada	3; 8; 5,27; 6,30	4
Czechoslovakia	3; 5; 6	
Denmark	3	4
Finland	9; 5	4, 1
France	3; 9; 6; 10,K; 14	4, 2, 1
Japan	3	
Nigeria	Untypable	1
South Africa	3; 5; 6	4, 1
Sweden	3; 9	
United States	8; Untypable; 5,27; 6; 5; 20	1, 2, 3, 4

the presence of lipase and DNAase. Most human isolates belong to Biotype 4, but Biotypes 1 and 2 have recently been recognized as potential human pathogens.

The large numbers of serotype and biotype combinations in *Y. enterocolitica* makes the identification of organisms complex. In epidemiological investigations, these antigenic and biochemical markers can be very useful for identifying pathogenic strains and tracing modes of transmission. In Table 3.6, there is a summary of some of the serotypes and biotypes that commonly have been identified in human cases in different geographic areas.

3.2.3. Reservoirs and Environmental Sources

Yersinia enterocolitica has been isolated in nature in many countries from a great diversity of animals, including livestock, dogs, cats, deer, monkeys, small mammals, and birds. However, the serotypes that are associated with human disease have been isolated infrequently from animals. In Europe, South Africa, Japan, and Canada, pigs have been found to be an important source of the human serotype O:3. The other human serotype O:9 has also been recovered from pigs, as well as from a dog and a cat. Table 3.7 shows some of the other possible animal sources of this infection, as well as some environmental sources.

TABLE 3.7
Animal and Environmental Sources of Human O Serotypes of *Yersinia enterocolitica*

Source	Serotypes	References
Pig	3; 3,5; 9	Ahvonen[86] Christensen[87] Mollaret[65] Toma and Deidrick[88] Toma[89] Wauters[90]
Cat	3; 9	Ahvonen[86] Toma[88,89]
Dog	20; 5,27; 3; 4; 9	Ahvonen[86] Toma[88,89] Tsubokura *et al.*[91] Wilson *et al.*[92]
Rat	5; 12; 20	Tsubokura *et al.*[91]
Oyster	5; 6,30	Toma[88,89]
Goose	4,33	Toma[88,89]
Beaver	Biotype 1	Toma[88,89]
Rabbit	2	Mollaret[65]
Chinchilla	1	Mollaret[65]
Stream water	8	Keet[63]
Well water	5; 4,33; 3; 18,28	Highsmith *et al.*[93]
Other water	5; 6,30; 6,31; 7,8	Caprioli *et al.*[94]
Chocolate milk	8	Black *et al.*[71]
Raw milk	5; 16; 10; 55	Hughes and Jensen[96] Vidon and Delmas[97] Schiemann and Toma[95]
Pasteurized milk	5a	Hughes[98]
Food, including ham, sausage, beef, cheese, pancake	4,32; 6,31	Caprioli *et al.*[94]

The importance of the pig as a natural reservoir of *Y. enterocolitica* in Europe has been stressed. Experimental infections of pigs by Wauters showed that the tonsils were culture-positive longer than were feces, suggesting that the oral cavity might be the source of human infection. Wauters[60] showed that over 50% of pigs' tongues cultured at Belgian butcher shops were culture-positive for *Y. enterocolitica,* serotype O:3 . Likewise, in Denmark Pedersen[61] showed that about 30% of the throat swabs of pigs taken to slaughter houses were positive for the same serotype.

The ascendant role of the pig in the epidemiology of yersiniosis has been questioned by Mollaret *et al.*[62] Their wide-ranging work in Europe has identified many animal reservoirs and environmental reservoirs, each of which contains a diversity of serotypes and biotypes. Foremost among these reservoirs are wild rodents, hares, chinchillas, and swine. They propose that certain strains are well adapted to certain reservoirs in which they exist and multiply and cause no disease. Man becomes sick when he is infected with certain strains which are not well adapted to man.

Additionally, isolations of *Y. enterocolitica* have been made from water. One of these was the American human serotype O:8 isolated from a stream in the Adirondack Mountains of New York.[63] River water in Wisconsin was examined by Meadows and Snudden,[64] who found that about 8% of 300 specimens were positive for *Y. enterocolitica*. Other strains have been isolated from well water or other water samples and from milk. Human fecal carriers who were asymptomatic or had recovered from an illness have been identified[65,66] and may be one source of the positive water samples.

An environmental feature of *Y. enterocolitica* infections in the United States is a tendency to occur in rural communities. Snyder *et al.*[67] showed that 30% of all *Y. enterocolitica* isolations were made in specimens from counties of Wisconsin with less than 30,000 people, whereas only 13% of all specimens submitted came from these small counties. It was suggested that rural inhabitants more frequently were in contact with uncooked meat and drank unpasteurized milk, to explain the increased susceptibility to infection.

Contaminated food may also be an important source of human infection. The organism has been found frequently in samples taken from swine slaughter-houses and also can be found in market meat and vacuum-packed beef.[68] It has been suggested by Fukushima *et al.*[69] that flies in kitchens or slaughter-houses can transfer infection to food; these workers actually cultured *Y. enterocolitica* from captured flies in Japan. The organism additionally has been isolated from ice cream, oysters, and mussels. The ability of *Y. enterocolitica* to grow at 4°C is the basis for the technique of cold enrichment of cultures (see Section 6.2.2) and could explain the potential hazard of infection from refrigerated meat.

3.2.4. Epidemics

In the United States at least four outbreaks of enteritis due to *Y. enterocolitica* have been defined. The first one occurred in 1973 in rural North

Carolina and affected 16 persons, of whom two died. There was a stepwise progression of illness through four neighboring families, suggesting interfamilial and person-to-person spread rather than a point source outbreak. Although the source was not located, a dog had just given birth to nine puppies, five of which died with diarrhea the week before the outbreak.(70) The second epidemic occurred in 1976 in upstate New York and resulted in the hospitalization of 36 children, 16 of whom had appendectomies. Infection was traced to contaminated chocolate milk served in schools. At the dairy that processed the milk, however, all cultures of milk and the environment were sterile, and it was suggested that contamination may have occurred when the milk and chocolate syrup were mixed by hand.(71) The third epidemic occurred in 1982 in Pennsylvania and affected 16 persons who attended a meeting of a Brownie Troop.(71a) Fifteen had abdominal symptoms including pain, diarrhea, and fever and three children underwent appendectomies. The median incubation period was 6 days. The source of infection was traced to bean sprouts that had been grown in refrigerated water obtained from a well that was shown to be contaminated by *Y. enterocolitica*. The fourth and largest epidemic occurred in 1982 causing infection in 172 persons in Tennessee, Arkansas, and Mississippi. Seventeen persons underwent appendectomies. Drinking pasteurized milk from a plant in Memphis, Tennessee, was associated with illness, but milk from the suspected lots was not available for culture.(71b)

Another outbreak of diarrhea at a ski resort in the United States was suspected to have been caused by *Y. enterocolitica* because it was isolated from water in the community. However, the organism was not cultured from the patients.(72) In Japan, well-defined outbreaks of *Y. enterocolitica* enteritis have been reported in both communities and schools.(73) At one junior high school in Japan in 1972, Zen-Yoji *et al.* reported that 198 pupils out of 1086 developed acute abdominal pain and fever.(66) Most cases occurred within a 3-day period, and there were no secondary cases among classmates, teachers, or families. Fecal specimens were positive for *Y. enterocolitica* serotype O:3 in the majority of patients during the illness. Follow-up fecal samples a month later remained positive in 19% of the patients. This outbreak suggested a single source of contaminated food or water, which was not identified, and the prolonged fecal carriage suggested the potential for secondary spread from the patients.

In Finland, the first hospital outbreak of *Y. enterocolitica* was reported in 1973 by Toivanen *et al.*(74) Approximately 10 days after a schoolgirl was admitted to a hospital with diarrhea, five staff members (four nurses and a cleaner) developed illnesses characterized by fever, abdominal pain, and diarrhea. Another nurse became ill later, after she worked with the ill members of the staff but not with the patient. Spread of the infection appeared to be from the patient to the staff and, then, person to person. Another hospital outbreak of *Y. enterocolitica* was reported from Newfoundland, Canada, in 1981 by Ratnam *et al.*[75] This involved nine patients and was diarrheal illness caused by an unusual strain of serotype O:5, Biotype 1. Some of the patients were in direct contact with hospital personnel. Most of the cases were elderly and had underlying medical diseases.

Spread of infection within families of children with diarrhea due to *Y. enterocolitica* serotype O:3 was shown by Marks *et al.* in Canada.[76] In 57 children, diarrhea lasted for a mean of 14 days. In their family contacts 8 of 117 adults (7%) and 12 of 41 children (29%) developed infections with culture-positive stools.

3.2.5. Seasonal Variation in Occurrence

No clear seasonal patterns of disease are apparent in the United States. Mollaret pointed out, however, that more cases occur in Europe during the autumn and winter (October–May) than during warmer seasons.[65] The seasonality of human disease can be correlated with the seasonality of isolations of *Y. enterocolitica* from pigs. Bockemühl *et al.*[77] showed that serotypes O:3 and O:9 were isolated from 2% of the pig feces in a German slaughterhouse. These human serotypes were isolated only in the months October to December, corresponding to the peak season for human infection.

This disease is also notable for its apparent rarity in tropical climates. This association of *Y. enterocolitica* infection with cooler seasons and the temperate climates of Europe, Canada, United States, Japan, and South Africa is consistent with the unique microbiological characteristics of *Y. enterocolitica* which include growth at 4°C and an optimal growth rate at 22–29°C.[68] Thus, the organism may be able to survive and even multiply in the environment after it has been passed from mammalian bodies in the feces. This temperature-dependent growth property could give *Y. enterocolitica* a competitive advantage over other bacteria for propagation in the environment.

3.2.6. Effects of Age and Sex

Children appear to be preferentially affected by *Y. entercolitica* infections. Children under 5 years usually developed mild gastroenteritis, whereas children over 5 years are more likely to develop the appendicitislike syndrome.[78] Mollaret reported that 168 of 359 infected patients (47%) were between one and five years old.[65] This propensity of infection for childhood may be similar to that of shigellosis, which is spread also by the fecal–oral route from person to person, and may simply reflect the less hygienic habits of children. Males have outnumbered females slightly in all age groups of patients with gastroenteritis, whereas the clinical syndrome of erythema nodosum has occurred more commonly in females.

3.2.7. Other Host Factors

Adults have a lower incidence of *Yersinia enterocolitica* infections because of, most probably, less exposure to contaminated environmental sources and greater immunity to infection that increases with age. On the other hand, Snyder *et al.*[67] demonstrated that persons with *Y. enterocolitica* infections in Wisconsin were more likely to have underlying medical diseases than were control subjects. The importance of host-immune factors in limiting the infection to the intestine is demonstrated also by the more frequent occurrence of bacteremia in adults with underlying diseases, including malignancies, liver diseases, hemolytic anemias, and hemochromatosis. There has also been a report of *Y. enterocolitica* bacteremia in an immunosuppressed patient, following renal transplantation.[79]

3.2.8. Relationship to Other Infections

3.2.8.1. *Salmonella*

Vandepitte and Wauters[50] showed that 8.5% of all stool specimens from persons with *Y. enterocolitica* had concomitant infections with *Salmonella* species, while only 4.3% of all stool specimens that were studied were positive for *Salmonella*. This higher-than-expected incidence of dual infections with *Yersinia* and *Salmonella* can be explained by the fact that both genuses have their reservoirs in farm animals and that humans who are exposed to one are exposed concomitantly to the other.

3.2.8.2. Plague

Mollaret and co-workers[62] have pointed out that geographical areas where plague occurs are usually free of *Y. enterocolitica* and vice versa. This exclusivity of two different *Yersinia* infections implies that infection with one genus may provide immunity against the other genus. Small mammals serve as reservoirs of both infections, and it is conceivable that cross-protective immunity keeps animal populations free of *Yersinia* infections. Experimental animal data will be further discussed in Chapter 7, Prevention and Control.

3.3. *YERSINIA PSEUDOTUBERCULOSIS* INFECTION

Yersinia pseudotuberculosis is the rarest of the three members of the genus *Yersinia* as a human pathogen. Nevertheless, it is a well-recognized animal pathogen and, like plague, it should be regarded as a zoonotic infection that only rarely and accidentally infects man. The list of animals that are naturally infected by this pathogen is extensive and includes guinea pigs, rabbits, deer, racoons, and diverse domestic and farm animals. Birds are also important reservoirs in nature in which epizootics occur; the organism frequently has been isolated from turkey, ducks, geese, pigeons, doves, pheasants, and canaries.[80]

Strains of *Y. pseudotuberculosis* are divided in six serologic groups that are designated as O groups I through VI. They are characterized by thermostable type-specific O antigens and thermolabile H antigen. All of these may produce human disease, but O groups I and II are the most commonly isolated groups from human specimens in England[81] and Germany.[82]

Since the 1950s this infection has been identified sporadically in European countries, including Germany, France, England, Norway, Finland, Czechoslovakia, and Hungary. Additionally, it has been diagnosed in North and South America, India, and Japan, suggesting a worldwide distribution.

In man the portal of entry is presumed to be the gastrointestinal tract, from which bacteria spread to cause acute mesenteric lymphadenitis or a generalized infection with septicemia. Persons with underlying cirrhosis of the liver appear to be particularly susceptible to the septicemic forms of this infection. In contrast to *Y. enterocolitica* infection, *Y. pseudotuberculosis* is rarely isolated from human feces and has not been demonstrated to cause diarrhea.

Males are affected about three times more frequently than females. The majority of patients have been children between 5–15 years old. Most patients developed illness in the winter with a peak incidence in November through February.[81] This seasonal pattern reflects the observed increased incidence of this infection in animals during the winter. Although there is no marked association of this disease with persons in intimate contact with animals, many patients that have been studied have been shown to have been in contact with an infected animal. Examples have included infected pet dogs,[82] as well as cats and canaries.[83] Family outbreaks have been reported,[84] but epidemiologic investigations have been inadequate to distinguish a common environmental source from intrafamilial spread of infection. No evidence exists for person-to-person spread of infection. As in other enteric infections of man that originate from animal reservoirs in nature, three possible modes of infection have been identified[81]: (1) direct contact with infected animals or their excreta, (2) ingestion of contaminated meat or other infected foodstuff, and (3) drinking contaminated water or milk. Well water in Czechoslovakia was recently shown by Aldova *et al.*[85] to be contaminated by *Y. pseudotuberculosis* Type II.

REFERENCES

1. Human plague in 1981, *Weekly Epidemiol. Rec.* **57:**289–291 (1982).
2. L. G. Lipson, Plague in San Francisco in 1900: The United States Marine Hospital Service Commission to study the existence of plague in San Francisco, *Ann. Intern. Med.* **77:**303–310 (1972).
3. M. Bahmanyar and D. C. Cavanaugh, *Plague Manual,* World Health Organization, Geneva (1976).
4. M. Baltazard, La conservation de la peste en foyer invertébré, *Med. Hyg. (Geneva)* **22:**172–174 (1964).
5. M. Baltazard and M. Bahmanyar, Recherches sur la peste en Inde, *Bull. W. H. O.* **23:**169–215, (1960).
6. B. Velimirovic, Plague in Southeast Asia: A brief historical summary and present geographical distribution, *Trans. R. Soc. Trop. Med. Hyg.* **66:**479–504 (1972).
7. B. Velimirovic, Review of the global epidemiological situation of plague since the last congress of tropical medicine and malaria in 1968, *Zentralbl. Bakteriol. Parasitenkd. Hyg. Infektionskr. Abt. Orig. Reihe A* **229:**127–133 (1974).
8. D. C. Cavanaugh, D. H. Hunter, N. V. Ba, T. C. Dung, P. F. Ryan, and J. D. Marshall, Ecology of plague in Vietnam III. Sylvatic plague; *Bandicota indica,* a transitional species, *Trans. R. Soc. Trop. Med. Hyg.* **62:**456 (1968).
9. J. D. Marshall, D. V. Quy, F. L. Gibson, T. C. Dung, and D. C. Cavanaugh, Ecology of plague in Vietnam: Commensal rodents and their fleas, *Mil. Med.* **132:**896–903 (1967).
10. J. D. Marshall, R. J. T. Joy, N. V. Ai, D. V. Quy, J. L. Gibson, and F. L. Gibson, Plague in Vietnam 1965–1965, *Am. J. Epidemiol.* **86:**603–616 (1967).
11. U. Thaung, K. M. Kyi, M. M. Sein, D. S. Myint, U. S. Win, R. Hein, and C. K. Ming, An outbreak of plague in Hlegu, Burma in 1977, *Southeast Asian J. Trop. Med. Public Health* **9:**390–397 (1978).

12. J. E. Brooks, U. H. Naing, D. W. Walton, D. S. Myint, U. M. M. Tun, U. Thaung and D. O. Kyi, Plague in small mammals and humans in Rangoon, Burma, *Southeast Asian J. Trop. Med. Public Health* **8:**335–344 (1977).
13. D. W. Walton and U. M. M. Tun, Fleas of small mammals from Rangoon, Burma, *Southeast Asian J. Trop. Med. Public Health* **9:**369–377 (1978).
14. A. Machiavello, Some special epidemiological and clinical features of plague in Northeastern Brazil, *Public Health Rep.* **56:**1657–1662 (1941).
15. C. R. Almeida, A. R. Almeida, J. B. Vieira, U. Guida, and T. Butler, Plague in northeast Brazil: Two years of bacteriological and serological surveillance, *Bull. W. H. O.* **59**(4)**:**591–597 (1981).
16. T. Butler, C. R. Almeida, A. R. Almeida, U. Guida, J. B. Vieira, A. Franco, and T. Quan, Estudos sorologicos e experimentais da peste no nordeste do Brasil, *Rev. Bras. Malariol. Doencas Trop.* **32:**26–35 (1980).
17. J. L. Caten and L. Kartman, Human plague in the United States 1900–1966, *J. Am. Med. Assoc.* **205:**333–336 (1968).
18. L. Kartman, Historical and ecological observations on plague in the United States, *Trop. Geogr. Med.* **22:**257–275 (1970).
19. D. L. Palmer, A. L. Kisch, R. C. Williams, and W. P. Reed, Clinical features of plague in the United States: The 1969–1970 epidemic, *J. Infect. Dis.* **124:**367–371 (1971).
20. B. W. Hudson, M. I. Goldenberg, J. D. McCluskie, H. E. Larson, C. D. McGuire, A. M. Barnes, and J. D. Poland, Serological and bacteriological investigations of an outbreak of plague in an urban tree squirrel population, *Am. J. Trop. Med. Hyg.* **20:**255–263 (1971).
21. *Morbidity and Mortality Weekly Report* **25:**155 (1976), **25:**253 (1976), **26:**215–216 (1977), **27:**259–260 (1978), **28:**285 (1979).
22. C. F. von Reyn, A. M. Barnes, N. S. Weber, and U. G. Hodgin, Bubonic plague from exposure to a rabbit: A documented case and a review of rabbit-associated cases in the United States, *Am. J. Epidemiol.* **104:**81–87 (1976).
23. C. F. von Reyn, A. M. Barnes, N. S. Weber, T. Quan, and W. J. Dean, Bubonic plague from direct exposure to a naturally infected wild coyote, *Am. J. Trop. Med. Hyg.* **25:**626–629 (1976).
24. C. F. von Reyn, N. S. Weber, B. Tempest, A. M. Barnes, J. D. Poland, J. M. Boyce, and V. Zalma, Epidemiologic and clinical features of an outbreak of bubonic plague in New Mexico, *J. Infect. Dis.* **136:**489–494 (1977).
25. J. D. Poland, A. M. Barnes, and J. J. Herman, Human bubonic plague from exposure to a naturally infected wild carnivore, *Am. J. Epidemiol.* **97:**332–337 (1973).
25a. H. Stark, Thesis for Master's Degree. Information obtained courtesy of Dr. T. J. Quan, Centers for Disease Control, Fort Collins, Colorado.
26. A. F. Kaufman, J. M. Boyce, and W. J. Martone, Trends in human plague in the United States, *J. Infect. Dis.* **141:**522–524 (1980).
27. J. M. Mann, W. J. Martone, J. M. Boyce, A. F. Kaufman, A. M. Barnes, and N. S. Weber, Endemic human plague in New Mexico: Risk factors associated with acquisition of infection, *J. Infect. Dis.* **140:**397–401 (1979).
28. J. E. Williams, B. W. Hudson, R. W. Turner, J. Sulianti Saroso, and D. C. Cavanaugh, Plague in Central Java, Indonesia, *Bull. W. H. O.* **58**(3)**:**459–468 (1980).
29. H. H. Mollaret, Conservation expérimentale de la peste dans le sol, *Bull. Soc. Pathol. Exot.* **56:**1168–1182 (1963).
30. L. Kartman, F. M. Prince, S. F. Quan, and H. E. Stark, New knowledge on the ecology of sylvatic plague. *Ann. N.Y. Acad. Sci.* **70:**668–711 (1958).
31. P. C. C. Garnham, Distribution of wild-rodent plague, *Bull. W. H. O.* **2:**271–278 (1949).

32. M. Baltazard and M. Bahmanyar, Recherches sur la peste à Java, *Bull. W. H. O.* **23:**217–246 (1960).
33. D. C. Cavanaugh, H. G. Dangerfield, D. H. Hunter, R. J. T. Joy, J. D. Marshall, D. V. Quy, S. Vivona, and P. E. Winter, Some observations on the current plague outbreak in the Republic of Vietnam, *Am. J. Public Health* **58:**742–752 (1968).
34. D. C. Cavanaugh, P. F. Ryan, and J. D. Marshall, The role of commensal rodents and their ectoparasites in the ecology and transmission of plague in Southeast Asia, *Bull. Wildlife Dis. Assoc.* **5:**187–194 (1969).
35. C. A. Green, D. H. Gordon, and N. F. Lyons, Biological species in *Praomys* (Mastomys) *natalensis* (Smith), a rodent carrier of Lassa virus and bubonic plague in Africa, *Am. J. Trop. Med. Hyg.* **27:**627–629 (1978).
36. M. Isaacson, L. Arntzen and P. Taylor, Susceptibility of members of the *Mastomys natalensis* species complex to experimental infection with *Yersinia pestis, J. Infect. Dis.* **144:**80 (1981).
37. S. C. Seal, Epidemiological studies of plague in India. 2. The changing pattern of rodents and fleas in Calcutta and other cities, *Bull. W. H. O.* **23:**293–300 (1960).
38. Suzuki and S. Hotta, Antiplague antibodies against *Yersinia pestis* Fraction I antigen in serum from rodents either experimentally infected or captured in harbor areas of Japan, 1971–1977, *Microbiol. Immunol.* **23**(12)**:**1157–1168 (1979).
39. A. W. Bacot, C. J. Martin, Observations on the mechanism of the transmission of plague by fleas, *J. Hyg.* **13:**432–439 (1914).
40. L. Kartman, Effects of differences in ambient temperature upon the fate of *Pasteurella pestis* in *Xenopsylla cheopis, Trans. R. Soc. Trop. Med. Hyg.* **63:**71–75 (1969).
41. D. C. Cavanaugh, Specific effect of temperature upon transmission of the plague bacillus by the oriental rat flea *Xenopsylla cheopis, Am. J. Trop. Med. Hyg.* **20:**264–273 (1971).
42. W. P. Olson, Rat-flea indices, rainfall, and plague outbreaks in Vietnam, with emphasis on the Pleiku area, *Am. J. Trop. Med. Hyg.* **18:**621–628 (1969).
43. J. H. Rust, D. C. Cavanaugh, R. O'Shita, and J. D. Marshall, The role of domestic animals in the epidemiology of plague. I. Experimental infection of dogs and cats, *J. Infect. Dis.* **124:**522–526 (1971).
43a. T. Butler, Y. S. Fu, L. Furman, C. Almeida, and A. Almeida, Experimental *Yersinia pestis* infection in rodents after intragastric inoculation and ingestion of bacteria, *Infect. Immun.*, **36:**1160–1167 (1982).
44. Y. Karimi, Conservation naturelle de la peste dans le sol, *Bull. Soc. Pathol. Exot.* **56:**1183–1186 (1963).
45. Y. Karimi, C. R. Almeida, and A. R. Almeida, La peste expérimentale chez les rongeurs du Brésil, *Bull. Soc. Pathol. Exot.* **67:**591–601 (1974).
46. J. D. Marshall, D. V. Quy, and F. L. Gibson, Asymptomatic pharyngeal plague infection in Vietnam, *Am. J. Trop. Med. Hyg.* **16:**175–177 (1967).
47. G. Blanc and M. Baltazard, Recherches sur le mode de transmission naturelle de la peste bubonique et septicémique. *Arch. Inst. Pasteur Maroc* **3:**175–354 (1945).
48. S. R. Ell, Some evidence for interhuman transmission of medieval plague, *Rev. Infect. Dis.* **1**(3)**:**563–566 (1979).
48a. A. K. Akiev, Epidemiology and incidence of plague in the world, 1958–1979, *Bull. W.H.O.* **60**(2)**:**165–169 (1982).
48b. J. B. Schleifstein and M. Coleman, An unidentified microorganism resembling *B. lignieri* and *Pasteurella pseudotuberculosis,* and pathogenic for man, *N.Y. State J. Med.* **39:**1749–1753 (1939).

49. E. J. Bottone, *Yersinia enterocolitica:* A panoramic view of a charismatic microorganism, *CRC Crit. Rev. Microbiol.* **5**:211–241 (1977).
50. J. Vandepitte and G. Wauters, Epidemiological and clinical aspects of human *Yersinia enterocolitica* infections in Belgium, *Contrib. Microbiol. Immunol.* **5**:150–158 (1979).
51. J. M. Alonso, H. Bercovier, J. Servan and H. H. Mollaret, Contribution to the study of the ecology of *Yersinia enterocolitica* in France, *Contrib. Microbiol. Immunol.* **5**:132–143 (1979).
52. A. Makulu, F. Gatti, H. H. Mollaret, and J. Vandepitte, Sur l'existence d'infections humaines à *Yersinia enterocolitica* en Republique du Congo, *Bull. Soc. Pathol. Exot.* **52**:452–460 (1969).
53. D. E. Agbonlahor, T. O. Odugbemi, and Q. Lasi, Isolation of *Yersinia enterocolitica* from stools of acute gastroenteritis cases in Lagos, Nigeria, *East Afr. Med. J.* **58**:520–524 (1981).
54. F. I. Anjorin, R. D. Sturrock, S. G. Subbuswamy, R. V. Lawande, and Y. M. Fakunle, *Yersinia enterocolitica* infection from West Africa: A case report, *Trans. R. Soc. Trop. Med. Hyg.* **73**:634–635 (1979).
55. A. C. Pizsolitto, D. P. Falcao, M. T. Shimizu, S. H. M. Galvao, and W. Giraldini, The first isolation of human *Yersinia enterocolitica* in Brazil: Case report, *Contrib. Microbiol. Immunol.* **5**:169–173 (1979).
56. E. Agner, M. Eriksen, H. Hollnagel, J. H. Larsen, H. I. Morck and M. Schroll, Prevalence of raised *Yersinia enterocolitica* antibody titre in unselected, adult populations in Denmark during 12 years, *Acta Med. Scand.* **209**:509–512 (1981).
57. R. Leino, Incidence of yersiniosis in Finland, *Scand. J. Infect. Dis.* **13**:309–310 (1981).
57a. M. L. Bissett, *Yersinia enterocolitica* from humans in California 1968–1975, *J. Clin. Microbiol.* **4**:137–144 (1976).
58. R. M. Robins-Browne, M. R. Jacobs, H. J. Koornhof, and A. C. Mauff, *Yersinia enterocolitica* biotype I in South Africa, *S. Afr. Medical J.* **55**:1057–1059 (1979).
59. G. Kapperud, *Yersinia enterocolitica* and *Y. enterocolitica*-like bacteria isolated from healthy humans in Norway, *Acta Pathol. Microbiol. Scand. Sect. B.* **88**:303–306 (1980).
60. G. Wauters, Carriage of *Yersinia enterocolitica* serotype 3 by pigs as a source of human infection, *Contrib. Microbiol. Immunol.* **5**:249–252 (1979).
61. K. B. Pedersen, Occurrence of *Yersinia enterocolitica* in the throat of swine, *Contrib. Microbiol. Immunol.* **5**:253–256 (1979).
62. H. H. Mollaret, H. Bercovier and J. M. Alonso, Summary of the data received at the WHO reference center for *Yersinia enterocolitica, Contrib. Microbiol. Immunol.* **5**:174–184 (1979).
63. E. E. Keet, *Yersinia enterocolitica* septicemia—source of infection and incubation period identified, *N.Y. State J. Med.* **74**:2226–2230 (1974).
64. C. A. Meadows, and B. H. Snudden, Prevalence of *Yersinia enterocolitica* in waters of the lower Chippewa River Basin, Wisconsin, *Appl. Environ. Microbiol.* **43**:953–954 (1982).
65. H. H. Mollaret, L'infection humaine à *Yersinia enterocolitica* en 1970 à la luminère de 642 cas récents, *Pathol. Biol.* **19**:189–205 (1971).
66. H. Zen-Yoji, T. Maruyama, S. Sakai, S. Kimura, T. Mizuno, and T. Momose, An outbreak of enteritis due to *Yersinia enterocolitica* occurring at a junior high school, *Jpn. J. Microbiol.* **17**:220–222 (1973).
67. J. D. Snyder, E. Christenson, and R. A. Feldman, Human *Yersinia enterocolitica* infections in Wisconsin: Clinical laboratory, and epidemiologic features, *Am. J. Med.* **72**:768–774 (1982).

68. G. K. Morris and J. C. Feeley, *Yersinia enterocolitica:* A review of its role in food hygiene, *Bull. W. H. O.* **54:**79–85 (1976).
69. H. Fukushima, Y. Ito, K. Saito, M. Tsubokura, and J. K. Otsuki, Role of the fly in the transport of *Yersinia enterocolitica, Appl. Environ. Microbiol.* **38:**1009–1010 (1979).
70. L. T. Gutman, E. A. Ottesen, T. J. Quan, P. S. Noce, and S. L. Katz, An inter-familial outbreak of *Yersinia enterocolitica* enteritis, *N. Engl. J. Med.* **288:**1372–1377 (1972).
71. R. E. Black, R. J. Jackson, T. Tsai, M. Medvesky, M. Shayegani, J. C. Feeley, K. I. E. Macleod, and A. M. Wakelee, Epidemic *Yersinia enterocolitica* infection due to contaminated chocolate milk, *N. Engl. J. Med.* **298:**76–79(1978).
71a. R. C. Aber, M. A. McCarthy, R. Berman, T. DeMelli, and E. White, An outbreak of *Yersinia enterocolitica* among members of a Brownie troop in Pennsylvania, *Program and Abstracts of the Twenty-Second Interscience Conference on Antimicrobial Agents and Chemotherapy,* Miami Beach, 1982, American Society for Microbiology (1982).
71b. Multi-state outbreak of yersiniosis, *Morbidity and Mortality Weekly Report* **31:**505–506 (1982).
72. K. V. Eden, M. L. Rosenberg, M. Stoopler, B. Wood, A. K. Highsmith, P. Skaliy, J. Wells, and J. C. Feeley, Waterborne gastroenteritis at a ski resort associated with the isolation of *Yersinia enterocolitica, Public Health Rep.* **92:**245–250 (1977).
73. Y. Asakawa, S. Akahane, N. Kagata, M. Noguchi, R. Sakazaki, and K. Tamura, Two community outbreaks of human infection with *Yersinia enterocolitica, J. Hyg.* **71:**715–723 (1973).
74. P. Toivanen, A. Toivanen, L. Olkkonen, and S. Aantaa, Hospital outbreak of *Yersinia enterocolitica* infection, *Lancet* **1:**801–803 (1973).
75. S. Ratnam, E. Mercer, B. Picco, and R. Butler, A nonsocomial outbreak of diarrheal disease due to *Yersinia enterocolitica* serotype O:5, biotype 1, *J. Infect. Dis.* **145:**242–247 (1982).
76. M. I. Marks, C. H. Pai, L. Laffeur, L. Lackman, and O. Hammerberg, *Yersinia enterocolitica* gastroenteritis: A prospective study of clinical, bacteriological, and epidemiologic features. *J. Pediatr.* **96:**26–31 (1980).
77. J. Bockemühl, H. Schmitt, J. Roth, and E. Saupe, Season-related incidence of *Yersinia enterocolitica* in fecal material of healthy slaughterhouse pigs, *Zentralbl. Bakteriol. Parasitenkd. Hyg. Infektionskr. Abt. Reihe Orig. A* **244:**494–505 (1979).
78. S. Kohl, *Yersinia enterocolitica* infections in children, *Pediatr. Clin North Am.* **26:**433–443 (1979).
79. J. Verhaegen, Y. Vanrenterghem, and J. Vandepitte, Generalized Yersinia enterocolitica infection in a renal transplant patient, *Infection* **9:**208–209 (1981).
80. T. N. Saari, and D. A. Triplett, *Yersinia pseudotuberculosis* mesenteric adenitis, J. Pediatr. **85:**655–659 (1974).
81. W. Knapp, Mesenteric adenitis due to *Pasteurella pseudotuberculosis* in young people, *N. Engl. J. Med.* **259:**776–778 (1958).
82. N. R. H. El-Maraghi and N. S. Mair, The histopathology of enteric infection with *Yersinia pseudotuberculosis, Am. J. Clin. Pathol.* **71:**631–639 (1979).
83. S. I. Hnatko and A. E. Rodin, *Pasteurella pseudotuberculosis* infection in man, *Can. Med. Assoc. J.* **88:**1108–1112 (1963).
84. K. J. Randall and N. S. Mair, Family outbreak of *Pasteurella pseudotuberculosis* infection, *Lancet* **1:**1042–1043 (1962).
85. E. Aldova, A. Brezinova, and J. Sobotkova, A finding of *Yersinia pseudotuberculosis* in well water, *Zentralbl. Bakteriol. Parasitenkd. Hyg. Infektionskr. Abt. Orig. Reihe B* **169:**265–270 (1979).

86. P. Ahvonen, Human yersiniosis in Finland. I. Bacteriology and serology, *Ann. Clin. Res.* **4**:30–38 (1972).
87. S. G. Christensen, *Yersinia enterocolitica* in Danish pigs *J. Appl. Bacteriol.* **48**(3):377–382 (1980).
88. S. Toma and V. R. Deidrick, Isolation of *Yersinia enterocolitica* from swine, *J. Clin. Microbiol.* **2**:478–481 (1975).
89. S. Toma, Survey on the incidence of *Yersinia enterocolitica* in the province of Ontario, *Can. J. Public Health* **54**:477–487 (1973).
90. G. L. Wauters, L. Le Minor, and A. M. Chalon, Antigènes somatiques et flagellaires des *Yersinia enterocolitica, Ann. Inst. Pasteur* **120**:631–642 (1971).
91. M. Tsubokura, T. Fukuda, K. Otsuki, M. Kubota, K. Itagaki, and S. Tanamachi, Isolation of *Yersinia enterocolitica* from some animals and meats, *Jap. J. Vet. Sci.* **37**:213–215 (1975).
92. H. D. Wilson, J. B. McCormick, and J. C. Feeley, *Yersinia enterocolitica* infection in a 4-month-old infant associated with infection in household dogs, *J. Pediatr.* **89**:767–769 (1976).
93. A. K. Highsmith, J. C. Feeley, P. Skaliy, J. G. Wells, and B. T. Wood, Isolation of *Yersinia enterocolitica* from well water and growth in distilled water, *Appl. Envir. Microbiol.* **34**:745–750 (1977).
94. T. Caprioli, A. J. Drapeau, and S. Kasatiya, *Yersinia enterocolitica:* Serotypes and biotypes isolated from human and the environment in Quebec, Canada, *J. Clin. Microbiol.* **8**:7–11 (1978).
95. D. A. Schiemann and S. Toma, Isolation of *Yersinia enterocolitica* from raw milk, *Appl. Envir. Microbiol.* **35**:54–58 (1978).
96. D. Hughes and N. Jensen, *Yersinia enterocolitica* in raw goat's milk, *Appl. Env. Microbiol.* **41**:309–310 (1981).
97. D. J. M. Vidon and C. L. Delmas, Incidence of *Yersinia enterocolitica* in raw milk in eastern France, *Appl. Env. Microbiol.* **41**:355–359 (1981).
98. D. Hughes, Repeated isolation of *Yersinia enterocolitica* from pasteurized milk in a holding vat at a dairy factory, *J. Appl. Bacteriol.* **48**:383–385 (1980).

4

Clinical Syndromes and Pathology in Humans

4.1. PLAGUE

4.1.1. Bubonic Plague

Although plague infection of man can assume many and protean clinical forms, the most common presentation, bubonic plague, in its typical clinical picture is so distinctive that both physicians and patients in endemic areas have little difficulty recognizing this disease. During an incubation period of 2–8 days following the bite of an infected flea, bacteria proliferate in the regional lymph nodes. Patients are typically affected by sudden onset of fever, chills, weakness, and headache. Usually at the same time, after a few hours, or on the next day, patients notice the bubo, which is signaled by intense pain in one anatomic region of lymph nodes, usually the groin, axilla, or neck. A swelling evolves in this area that is so tender that the patients typically avoid any motion that would provoke tenderness of the affected lymph nodes. For example, if the bubo is in a femoral area, the patients will characteristically flex, abduct, and externally rotate the hip to relieve pressure on the area and will walk with a limp. When the bubo is in an axilla, the patients will abduct the shoulder or hold the arm in a splint. When a bubo is cervical in location, patients will tilt their heads to the opposite side. This extreme tenderness of the buboes naturally causes patients to resist physicians' attempts to palpate and aspirate their buboes.

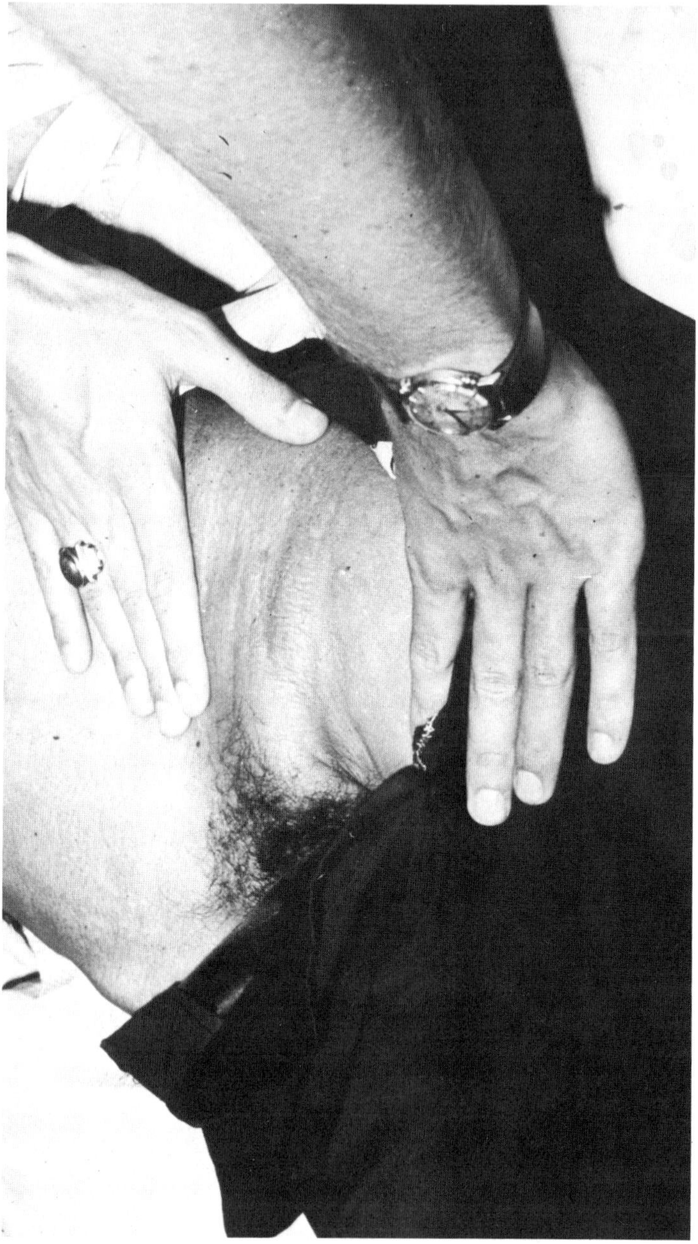

Figure 4.1. A left inguinal bubo consisting of a cluster of lymph nodes with overlying erythema of the skin and edema extending medially. Smaller secondary lymph nodes are present below in the femoral area.

The buboes of patients with plague are oval swellings varying from about 1 to 10 cm in length and elevate the overlying skin, which may appear stretched or erythematous. They may appear either as a smooth, uniform egg-shaped mass or as an irregular cluster of several lymph nodes with intervening and surrounding edema. Palpation will typically elicit extreme tenderness. There is warmth of the overlying skin and an underlying firm, nonfluctuant mass. Usually around the lymph nodes there is considerable edema which can be either gelatinous or pitting in nature. Occasionally, there is a large area of edema extending from the bubo into the skin region which is drained by the affected lymph nodes (see Figures 4.1 and 4.2).

Infections other than plague can produce acute lymphadenitis. Plague is, however, virtually unique for the suddenness of onset of the fever and bubo, the rapid development of intense inflammation in the bubo, and the fulminant clinical course which can produce death as quickly as from 2 to 4 days after the onset of symptoms. The bubo of plague is also distinctive for the usual absence of a detectable skin lesion in the anatomic region of the bubo and likewise for the absence of an ascending lymphangitis near the bubo.

The groin is the most common site of the buboes in plague. When clinical reports have distinguished femoral from inguinal locations, the femoral site is most frequent. Other common sites are the axillae and cervical region as shown in Table 4.1. The reason for a given distribution of buboes is presumed to be the distribution of flea bites through which the bacteria are inoculated into the skin and then migrate to the regional lymph nodes. The series of Burkle[1] contained a high percentage of cervical buboes in young children, whereas Butler[2] and Thuat and Tiep[3] predominantly reported adults, who had fewer cervical nodes. This difference suggests that adults, who more often are standing, are bitten by fleas on the legs, whereas children playing on the ground are more likely to get flea bites on the head or neck.

In uncomplicated bubonic plague, the patients are typically prostrate and lethargic and often exhibit restlessness or agitation. Occasionally they are delirious with high fever, and seizures are common in children. Temperatures are usually elevated, in the range 38.5 to 40.0°C, and the pulse rates are increased to 110–140/min. Blood pressures are characteristically low, about 100/60 mm Hg, due to extreme vasodilation. Lower pressures that are unobtainable may occur if shock ensues. The liver and spleen are often palpable and tender.

All of these clinical features of bubonic plague have been known for centuries by physicians dealing with this disease. In the United States bubonic

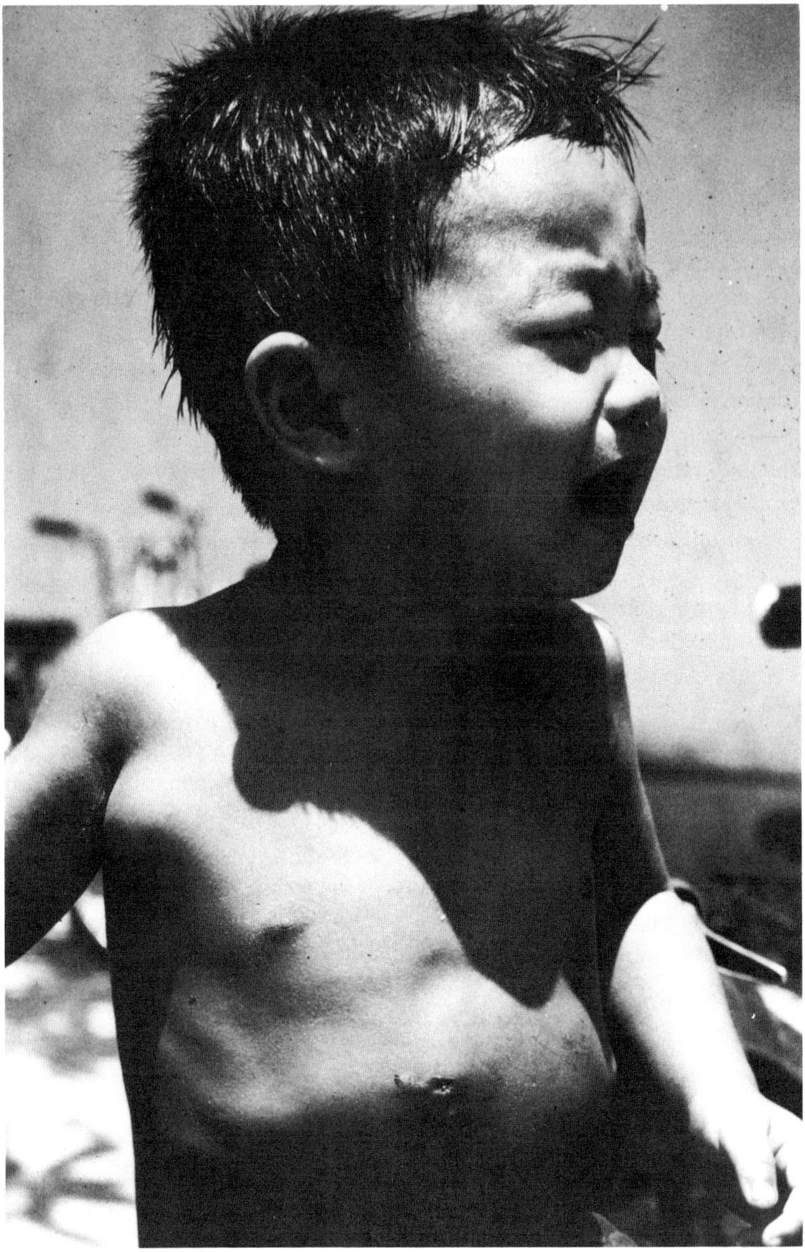

Figure 4.2. A left axillary bubo is very sensitive to motion of the arm. Skin of abdomen shows ulcer of presumed flea-bite site.

TABLE 4.1
Anatomic Distribution of Buboes in Three Series of Plague Reported from Vietnam

	Percent of patients with buboes in each region				
	Femoral and/or inguinal	Femoral	Inguinal	Axillary	Cervical
Thuat and Tiep[3] (500 cases)	60	Not stated		16	8
Burkle[1] (88 cases)	52	Not stated		9	33
Butler[2] (40 cases)	86	65	23	15	5

plague first occurred in San Francisco in 1900 and the clinical features of six cases were lucidly described by L. F. Barker.[4] American physicians in Vietnam from 1965 to 1975 were given opportunities to rediscover the dramatic clinical presentations of plague, and I have cited several of these reports[5–8] as well as the continuing flow of case reports in the United States that document the resurgence of plague in this country during the last decade.[9]

The pathology of bubonic plague was amply detailed by Simon Flexner in 1901.[10] The buboes consisted of unmistakable pathology, characterized by hemorrhage and necrosis. The border of the lymph nodes that is usually defined by the capsule was obliterated by the destructive inflammatory process which involved the periglandular tissues as much as the lymph nodes themselves. The normal architecture that separated cortex from medulla was destroyed. The lymphoid cells of the medulla were all necrotic. There were large phagocytic cells, polymorphonuclear leukocytes, red cells, and a granular material that appeared to be a pure culture of plague bacilli. Blood vessels were thrombosed. The bacteria existed in large numbers in both glandular and periglandular tissues. Flexner wrote, "In no known bacterial infectious process, not even in leprosy, are such large numbers of bacteria to be found. They occur in continuous growth throughout the glands, occupying every available space; they completely occlude many blood vessels, or, mixed with definite thrombi, compose a considerable part of the plugs. . . . The blood vessels and lymph vessels in the periglandular structures are also, to a large extent, occupied by bacilli. . . ."[10] This massive concentration of *Yersinia pestis* in the buboes allows one to make the diagnosis readily by the bubo aspirate and smear (Figure 4.3). In the early stage of disease the bubo does

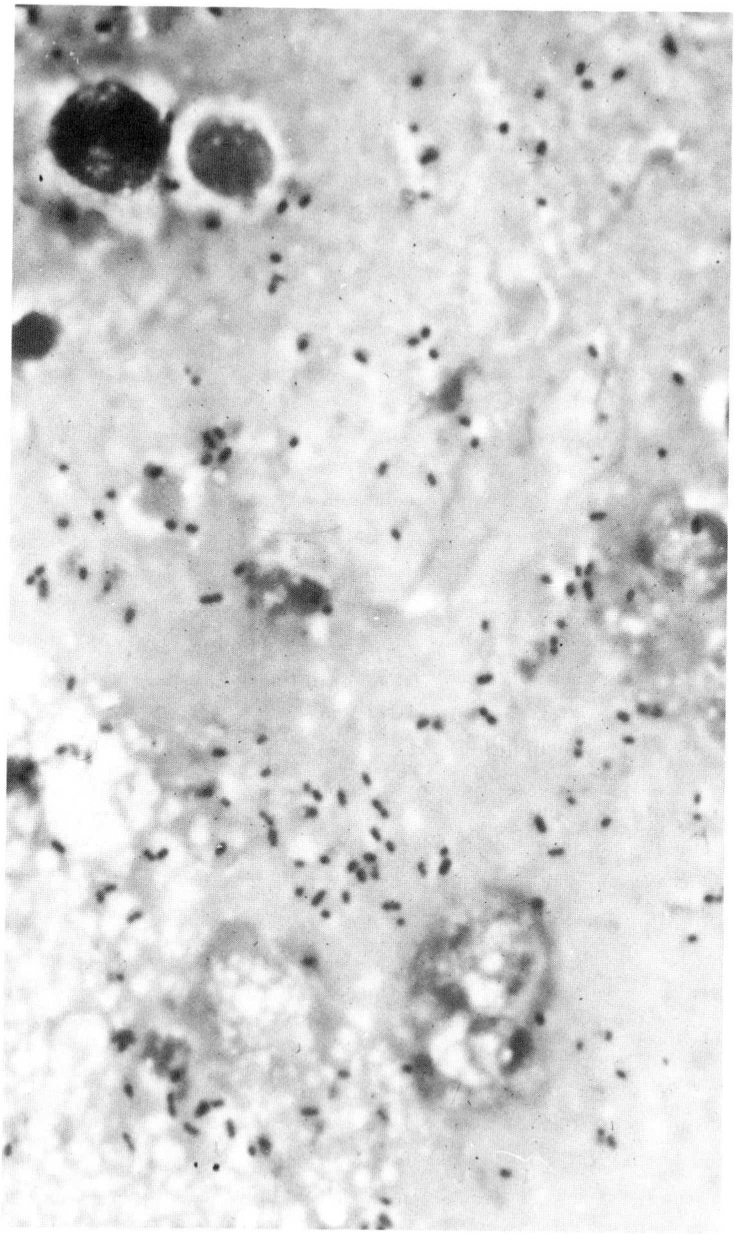

Figure 4.3. A bubo aspirate from a patient was smeared. The slide stained with Wayson's stain revealed bacilli that were pleomorphic and often bipolar.

not contain liquid pus. Accordingly, needle aspiration yields scanty serosanguinous fluid, and saline may have to be injected and reaspirated to obtain material for diagnosis.

Two recently described features of plague buboes are worthy of mention. Stahly and Shoop reported that a radioactive gallium scan in a patient with plague showed a large area of increased uptake of the isotope in the area of the axillary bubo, as well as increased uptake by the meninges when the patient developed meningitis as a complication.(11) In Vietnam, Thuat and Tiep(3) and Dr. K. Arnold (personal communication) reported another new finding of subcutaneous emphysema near the buboes of some patients with plague. Whether the gas was introduced during the needle aspiration of the bubo or was gas produced by superinfecting bacteria of the bubo could not be determined, but this newly recognized feature of plague buboes requires confirmation by future observations.

4.1.2. Cutaneous Manifestations

The majority of patients with bubonic plague do not have skin lesions. About a fourth of the patients in Vietnam, however, did show varied skin findings.(2) The most common were pustules, vesicles, eschars, or papules near the bubo or in the anatomic region of skin that is drained lymphatically by the affected lymph nodes (Figures 4.4 and 4.5). These were presumably sites of the flea-bite inoculations. When opened, these lesions usually contained white cells and plague bacilli. Rarely, these skin lesions progress to produce extensive cellulitis or abscesses. Ulceration may lead, however, to a larger plague carbuncle. A neonatal patient in the United States was recently reported by White *et al.*(12) to have presented with a hemorrhagic macule surrounded by erythema on the knee; there was no adenopathy but the skin lesion and blood culture were positive for *Y. pestis*.

Another kind of skin lesion in plague is purpura, which has nothing to do with inoculation of the bacteria, but is a result of the systemic disease. The purpura may become necrotic, resulting in gangrene of distal extremities that is the probable basis of the epithet "black death" which has been attributed to plague through the ages. Although this is a rare complication of plague, Butler observed it in 2 of 40 cases in Vietnam,(2) and Stockard reported it in four other cases as a late complication in convalescing patients.(13) Purpuric lesions on the legs of two patients in the acute stage of bubonic plague were biopsied. Both showed cutaneous hemorrhage and necrosis and blood vessels

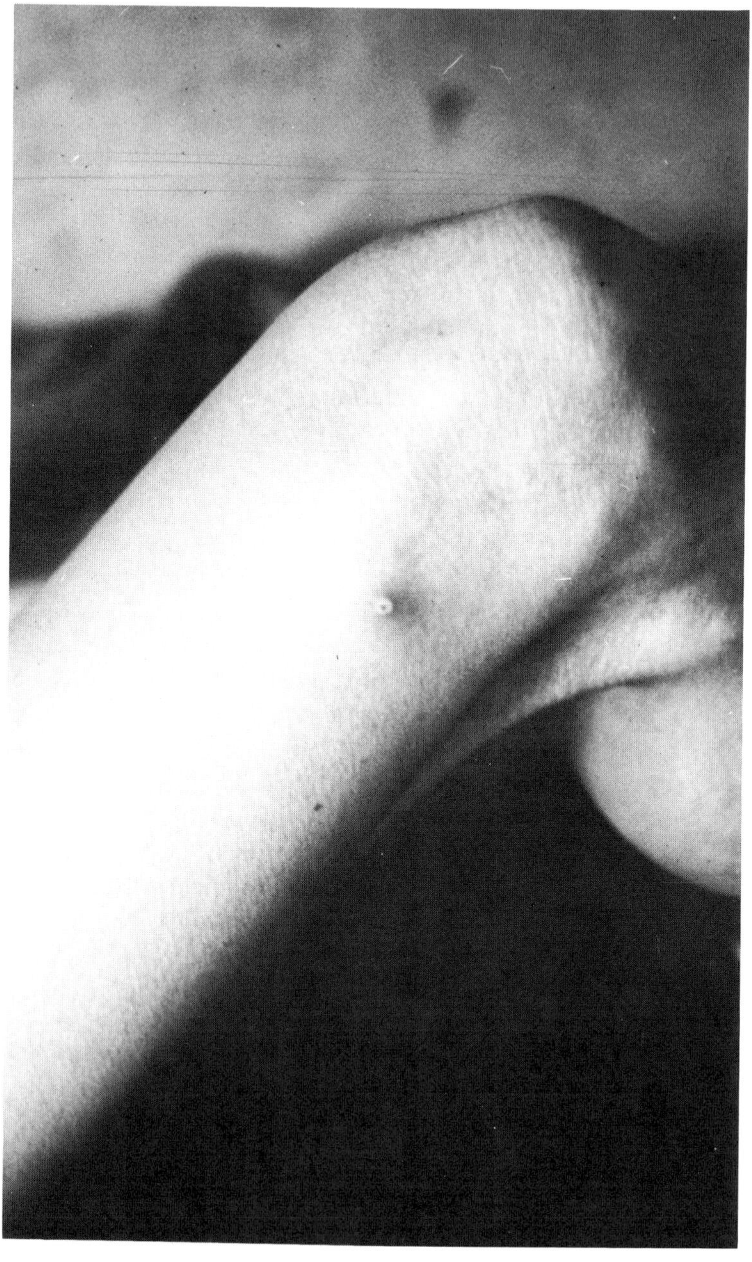

Figure 4.4. A pustule surrounded by erythema on the right thigh of a patient with a right femoral bubo. Both the pustule and bubo aspirate yielded a culture of *Y. pestis*.

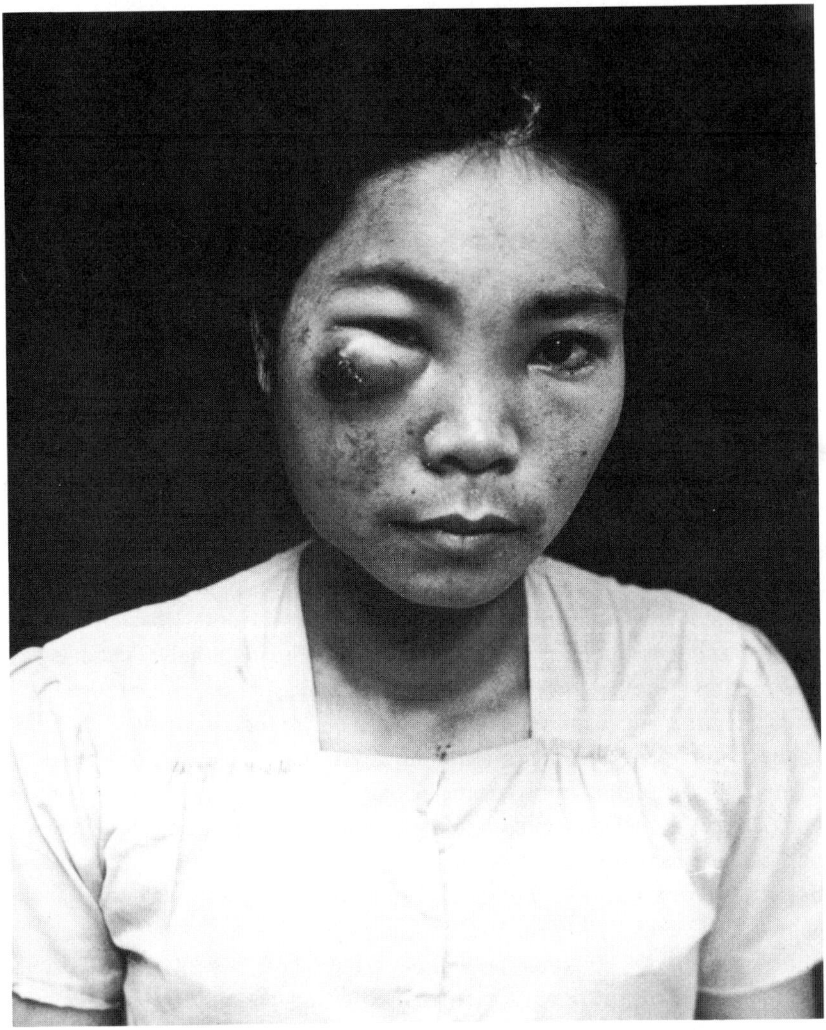

Figure 4.5. A subcutaneous abscess with overlying eschar below the right eye of a patient who also had a right submandibular bubo. Both pus from the abscess and a bubo aspirate yielded cultures of *Y. pestis*.

showed vasculitis and occlusion by fibrin thrombi. This lesion resembles the local Shwartzman reaction in rabbits that is produced by an intradermal injection of endotoxin followed the next day by an intravenous injection of endotoxin. Accordingly, this necrotic purpura of plague has been attributed to an action of endotoxin from *Y. pestis*.[14–15]

4.1.3. Septicemic Plague

A distinctive feature of plague, in addition to the bubo, is the propensity of the disease to overwhelm patients with a massive growth of bacteria in the blood. In the early acute stages of bubonic plague, all patients probably have intermittent bacteremia. Single blood cultures obtained at the time of hospital admission in Vietnamese patients were positive in 28 of 104 patients, or 27%.[2,15–17] In one of these studies,[17] 11 of 42 patients with bubonic plague had $\geqslant 10^2$ bacteria/ml of blood and were shown to have lower blood pressures and a higher mortality rate (27%) than patients with fewer bacteria or negative cultures (3%). A hallmark of moribund patients with plague is high-density bacteremia, so that a blood smear revealing characteristic bacilli has been used as a prognostic indicator in this disease. I have seen only one patient of eight with a positive blood smear for bacilli survive his infection.

Occasionally in the pathogenesis of plague infection, bacteria are inoculated and proliferate in the body without producing a bubo. Patients may become ill with fever and actually die with bacteremia but without detectable lymphadenitis. This syndrome has been termed "septicemic plague" to denote plague without a bubo. This term, however, has given rise to confusion, because most patients with bubonic plague have bacteremia at some time in their clinical evolution, and some authors have called bubonic plague with high-density bacteremia "septicemic" or "bubonic–septicemic." Septicemic plague has been noted to have a higher mortality rate than bubonic plague, as high as 27% and 100% in Vietnamese experiences.[3,5] The reason for the higher mortality is, in part, that without a bubo both patients and physicians fail to recognize the gravity of the disease and patients suffer a delay in receiving appropriate antibiotics.

4.1.4. Pneumonic Plague

One of the feared complications of bubonic plague is secondary pneumonia. The infection reaches the lungs by hematogenous spread of bacteria from the bubo. In addition to the high mortality, plague pneumonia is highly contagious by airborne transmission. The patient presents with fever and lymphadenopathy as cough, chest pain, and often, hemoptysis. Radiographically, there is patchy bronchopneumonia or confluent consolidation. The sputum is usually purulent and contains plague bacilli.

Primary inhalation pneumonia is rare now, but is a potential threat following exposure to a patient with plague who has a cough. It can be so rapidly fatal that persons reportedly have been exposed, became ill, and died on the same day. Plague pneumonia is invariably fatal when antibiotic therapy is delayed more than 20 hr after the onset of illness.[18]

Plague pneumonia appears to be a rare complication of bubonic plague, as larger series of patients in Vietnam reported only from 0 to 3% of patients to have pneumonia.[2,5] Furthermore, the three patients with signs of pneumonia in Butler's series[2] did not have positive sputum cultures for *Y. pestis* and, therefore, may have had other causes for pneumonia. Nevertheless, there were reports of both primary and secondary pneumonic plague in Vietnam verified by sputum culture.[6,8,19] Two case reports of pneumonia were described in American patients in Vietnam, one with primary pneumonia without a bubo[20] and one secondary case with a bubo.[6] Both patients survived. There was no airborne spread of infection from these cases, but another report of an outbreak of mixed pneumonic and bubonic plague suggested that person-to-person dissemination of primary pneumonia did occur in Vietnam.[19]

In the United States, secondary pneumonia in bubonic plague appears to be relatively more common. During 1975–1976, when there was a total of 36 cases of plague in the country, evidence was found for pneumonia in eight patients, or 22% (J. D. Poland, personal communication). All had pulmonary infiltrates in the setting of bubonic plague and seven of them had *Y. pestis* demonstrated in their sputum. Four patients (50%) died. Three of them died only 1 day after the recognition of the pneumonia but 5–7 days after the onset of the other symptoms of plague. These patients died despite appropriate antibiotic treatment, showing how fulminant this disease can be. There were no secondary cases of pneumonia among the contacts of these patients.

4.1.5. Meningeal Plague

Plague meningitis typically occurs more than a week following inadequately treated bubonic plague. It results from hematogenous spread from a bubo and carries a high mortality rate when compared with uncomplicated bubonic plague. Less commonly, plague meningitis presents as a primary infection of the meninges without antecedent lymphadenitis. Plague meningitis is characterized by fever, headache, meningismus, and spinal fluid pleocytosis with a predominance of polymorphonuclear leukocytes. Bacteria are frequently demonstrable with a gram stain of spinal fluid sediment, and endotoxin has been demonstrated in spinal fluid with the limulus test.[(17)]

When three patients with plague meningitis in Vietnam presented with a history of recently treated bubonic plague with their buboes in the axillary location, I reviewed the literature to find reported cases of plague meningitis where there was co-existing bubonic plague and information on the location of the bubo. Out of the 32 cases shown in Table 4.2, 20 patients or 63% of the total had axillary buboes. This association is remarkable when we consider that the majority of buboes in plague are femoral and inguinal. Possible reasons for this association have been speculated to be that more proximate lymphatic communications exist between axillary lymph nodes and the meninges.[(17)] Alternatively, von Reyn[(21)] has suggested that axillary plague often results from persons directly handling infected animal tissues, whereas femoral and inguinal plagues result from flea bites. Plague bacilli in animal tissues at 37°C have an antiphagocytic capsule and are more virulent than bacteria growing at lower ambient temperatures in the flea. This greater virulence of the bacteria

TABLE 4.2
Patients with Plague Meningitis in Which the Bubo Location Was Specified

No. of patients	No. with axillary bubo	No. deaths	Reference
7	3	6	Meyer *et al.*, 1937[(86)]
2	2	2	Koenigsfeld and Nambiar, 1946[(87)]
7	4	6	Landsborough and Tunnell, 1947[(88)]
1	0	0	Feeley and Kriz, 1965[(89)]
2	1	0	Martin *et al.*, 1967[(90)]
1	1	0	Reed *et al.*, 1970[(9)]
2	1	0	Tuan *et al.*, 1970, 1971[(91,92)]
2	1	0	Isaacson *et al.*, 1973[(93)]
2	2	1	Cantey, 1974[(5)]
1	1	0	Brown, 1974 (unpublished)
1	1	0	von Reyn *et al.*, 1976[(95)]
3	3	1	Butler *et al.*, 1976[(17)]
1	0	1	von Reyn *et al.*, 1977[(21)]
TOTALS 32	20	17	

in animal tissues or a larger average inoculum size from handling animals might explain this greater likelihood of developing meningitis.

4.1.6. Plague Pharyngitis

Plague can produce pharyngitis that may resemble acute tonsillitis. The anterior cervical lymph nodes are usually inflamed, and *Y. pestis* may be recovered from throat culture or aspiration of a cervical bubo. This is a rare clinical form of plague which is presumed to follow the inhalation or ingestion of plague bacilli. Asymptomatic pharyngeal infection was also described in Vietnam.(22) In some cultures, plague pharyngitis has been noted predominantly in women and has been related to their practice of grooming each others' hair for lice or fleas that are killed by biting them between their teeth.

4.1.7. Liver and Spleen Involvement

Although the liver and spleen are not primary target organs in plague infection, hematogenous spread of bacteria leads to infection of these and other organs. The liver is frequently enlarged, and liver function tests typically show mildly elevated blood enzyme levels and bilirubin concentrations. Patients are rarely jaundiced, however, as the highest bilirubin in our series of 10 patients was 2.4 mg/100 ml.(15) The most severely ill patients with high fever and delirium tended to have greater degrees of liver dysfunction; one fatal case in our series had a serum glutamic-oxaloacetic acid transminase of 300 units/ml just before death.

Liver dysfunction in a febrile comatose patient with hypoglycemia caused physicians in the United States recently to make an initial diagnosis of Reye's syndrome. The correct diagnosis of septicemic plague was revealed by blood culture and a history of the patient skinning rabbits; four days after admission he developed an axillary bubo.(23)

Another patient with bubonic plague developed liver dysfunction and a liver biopsy obtained about 2 months after the onset of his illness showed granulomatous inflammation.(24) Thus, plague infection may involve the liver in a variety of clinical forms.

Clinically detectable splenomegaly occurs only rarely in patients with bubonic plague. Nevertheless, the spleen is affected by this bacteremic infection and autopsies of plague victims have revealed spleens to be about twice the normal size.[10] The reasons for the usual absence of clinical splenomegaly may be that the suddenness of the disease evolution does not allow time for the spleen to enlarge greatly and that palpation of the abdomen is an insensitive test for splenomegaly.

The pathologic changes that are present in the liver and spleen confirm that these organs both are altered during plague infection. The liver typically shows no gross pathology, but microscopically there are bacilli and a diffuse increase of polymorphonuclear leukocytes in the sinusoids.[25] Flexner described the spleen as being congested and containing large numbers of plague bacilli and phagocytic cells.[10] Finegold reported that the sinusoids were depleted of cells and contained granular material which resembled fibrin, and there were foci of lymphoid necrosis.[25]

4.1.8. Kidney Involvement

The kidneys are not affected directly by infection during the course of acute bubonic plague. The urine may be concentrated because of fever and dehydration, and the blood urea nitrogen is transiently elevated out of proportion to the serum creatinine. There is occasionally proteinuria. In fatal cases of plague, however, Finegold reported that autopsies of four of eight patients showed fibrin thrombi in the glomerular capillaries.[25] This resembled the renal lesion of the generalized Shwartzman reaction in rabbits given two intravenous injections of endotoxin at an interval of 24 hr; after the second injection the rabbits develop anuria and intravascular coagulation and die with renal cortical necrosis and occlusive fibrin thrombi in many organs, as well as in the kidneys. This renal lesion of human plague led Finegold to postulate that plague may be fatal because of an endotoxemia that deposits fibrin in the vessels of the kidney and other organs.

4.1.9. Cardiac Involvement

Like the kidney, the heart is not a target organ for the infection, and there are no reports in the literature of serious cardiac involvement such as myocardial abscesses or endocarditis. Nevertheless, certain cardiac abnormalities may occur in bubonic plague. Patients typically have tachycardia, in the range of 100–140 cycles/min, that accompanies the fever. Older adults, however, frequently have lower pulse rates in the normal range, despite elevated temperatures.[16]

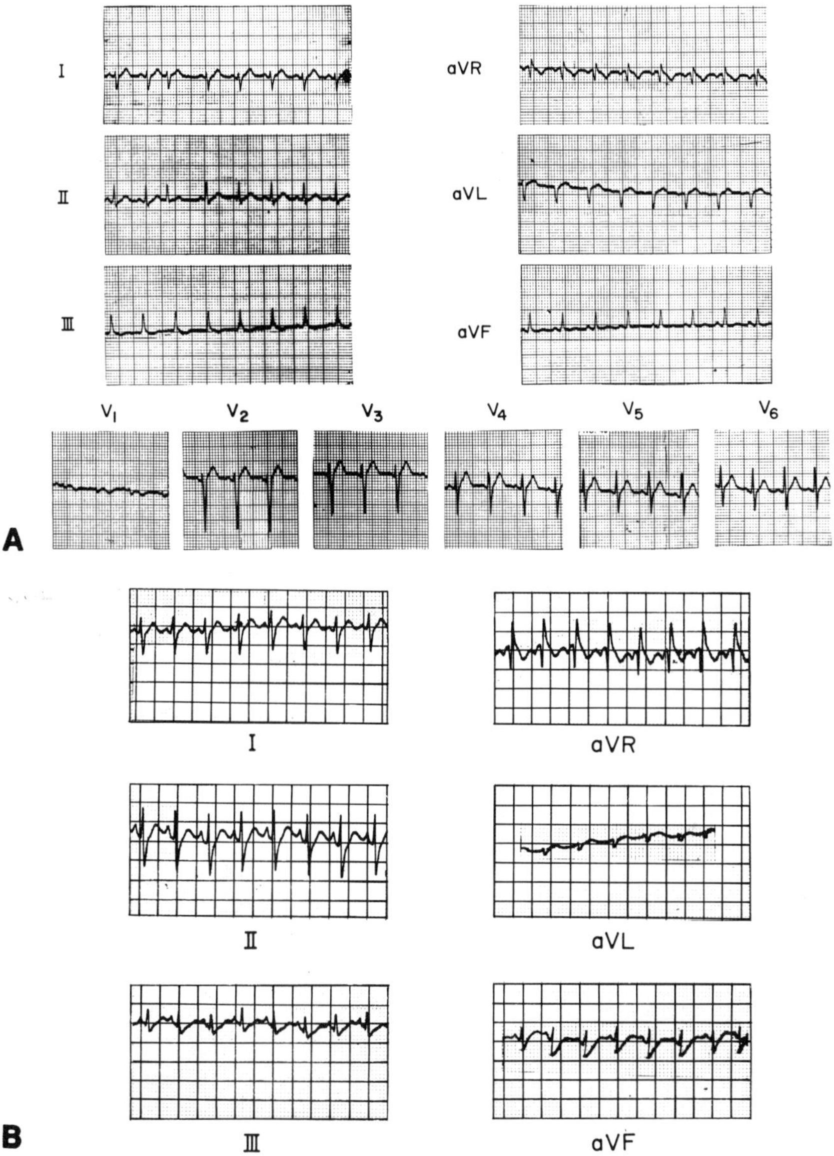

Figure 4.6. Electrocardiograms of patients with acute plague. (A) A 35-year-old woman with a pulse rate of 170/min showed sinus tachycardia and ST-segment depression indicative of myocardial ischemia. She died the same day. (B) Electrocardiogram of a 16-year-old girl with bubonic plague showed a sinus tachycardia with a ventricular rate of 135/min, frequent premature atrial contractions, right axis deviation + 120°, and a delayed precordial transition.

Electrocardiograms have revealed most commonly sinus tachycardia without other electrical abnormality. Some patients showed ST-T wave changes, such as ST-segment depression, that indicated cardiac ischemia had been caused by the tachycardia. In other patients, premature atrial contractions have been shown, as well as tall P waves and right axis deviation (Figure 4.6). These changes were interpreted as suggestive of acute cor pulmonale, which could have resulted from elevated pressures in the pulmonary arteries secondary to arterial vasoconstriction.[(2)] None of these patients, however, had other clinical signs of pulmonary involvement.

4.1.10. Hematological Aspects

Plague infection does not directly affect the red cells or hemoglobin concentration. Many patients with plague, however, show anemia probably because of preexisting nutritional or iron deficiencies. The white blood cell count is typically elevated in the range of 10,000–20,000 cells/mm^3, with a predominance of immature and mature neutrophils. The patients who appear most severely ill tend to have the higher white blood cell counts. Occasionally, some patients, especially children, may develop myelocytic leukemoid reactions with white cell counts as high as 100,000/mm^3.[(2)] Examination of the white blood cells in the peripheral blood smear typically reveals the so-called toxic changes of cytoplasmic vacuolations, toxic granulations, and Döhle's inclusion bodies that are characteristic of acute bacterial infections. Blood eosinophils are characteristically diminished or absent in the acute stage of infection, but return to normal or elevated levels during convalescence.

Blood platelets may be normal or low in the early stages of bubonic plague. In one study of 22 patients with plague, the mean platelet count was 180,000/mm^3. Six of these patients had platelet counts of less than 100,000/mm^3, indicative of clinically significant thrombocytopenia. Although patients with plague rarely develop a generalized bleeding tendency from profound thrombocytopenia, Butler *et al.* have established that disseminated intravascular coagulation (DIC) is common in this infection.[(16)] The clinical definition of DIC consists of (1) a reduction of platelets due to their entrapment in intravascular clots, (2) consumption of fibrinogen and other clotting factors which results in prolonged prothrombin and partial thromboplastin times, and (3) the generation of the degradation products fibrinogen and fibrin due to activation of thrombolytic enzymes. Patients with plague occasionally show these abnormalities of blood clotting. The most specific of these tests for DIC is the presence of fibrinogen–fibrin degradation products, which were detected in elevated titers in 19 of 22 patients who were tested in Vietnam. In these same patients decreased fibrinogen concentrations were found in only six patients and platelets less than 150,000/mm^3 in only seven patients (Table 4.3). The normal levels of fibrinogen that were found in most patients, despite other evidence for a consumption of this protein during DIC, may be explained by an increased production of fibrinogen which is known to occur in many inflammatory conditions. These blood findings of intravascular coagulation

TABLE 4.3
Tests for Disseminated Intravascular Coagulation in Patients with *Yersinia pestis* Infection on Admission to the Hospital and during Convalescence[a]

	Admission			Convalescence		
Patient No.	Platelets/mm^3	Fibrinogen (mg/100 ml)	FDP–fdp (titer)[b]	Platelets	Fibrinogen (mg/100 ml)	FDP–fdp (titer)
1	364,000	135	8			
2	190,000	360	8			
3	222,000	285	16	250,000	170	8
4	298,000	540	64	574,000	340	32
5	301,000	250	32	486,000	145	16
6	114,000	85	16	242,000	99	8
7	78,000	310	8	274,000	170	4
8	198,000	270	8			
9	200,000	270	128			
10	82,000	300	32	366,000	500	4
11	152,000	340	8	134,000	285	2
12	74,000	300	8	106,000	600	8
13	64,000	105[c]	256	200,000	210	4
14	178,000	270	32	184,000	270[c]	64
15	62,000	140	32	174,000	105[c]	—
16	284,000	300	2	270,000	300[c]	4
17	156,000	300	8	310,000	340	8
18	64,000	540	64	116,000	300	32
19	198,000	190	8	428,000	220[c]	64
20	150,000	340[c]	4	250,000	300	4
21	208,000	540[c]	2	216,000	250	2
22	312,000	135	64	366,000	80	32
Means[d]	180,000	287	16.6	275,000	260	9.5

[a] Adapted from Butler *et al.*[16] with permission of publisher.
[b] (FDP–fdp) Fibrinogen–fibrin degradation products. Normal titers are 4.
[c] Fibrinogen concentration measured may be lower than actual value because of a clot that formed in the citrate solution. Normal range is 250–400 mg/100 ml.
[d] Arithmetic means of platelets and fibrinogen; geometric means of FDP–fdp titers.

can be related pathophysiologically to the purpuric skin lesions of some patients that contain fibrin thrombi within the dermal blood vessels.[2]

4.1.11. Plague-Simulating Surgical Emergencies

Since plague may affect lymph nodes in any location, it must be considered in the differential diagnosis of all cases of suppurative adenitis. Inguinal or iliofemoral lymphadenopathies have been mistaken for strangulated hernias. Similarly, lymphadenopathy affecting iliofemoral paraaortic or retroperitoneal nodes has resulted in laparotomy for mistaken acute surgical abdomen. Some of these diagnostic errors can be avoided by appreciating that fever and the other constitutional symptoms characteristic of plague usually precede the lymphadenitis by a few hours or days.

4.1.12. Differential Diagnosis

Although bubonic plague presents a typical clinical picture that allows the diagnosis to be readily made in most cases, other acute infections can simulate plague. In the United States, an important infection that mimics plague is tularemia.[14,26] This infection has a similar clinical picture of fever and bubo, but has other epidemiological and clinical characteristics that assist physicians in distinguishing them (Table 4.4).

When buboes are present in the inguinal region, several venereal infections are considered. These include secondary syphilis, lymphogranuloma venereum, granuloma inguinale, and chancroid. When acute lymphadenitis develops in any anatomic location, the common bacterial infections which are due to *Staphylococcus aureus* and *Streptococcus pyogenes* are suspected; skin lesions of cellulitis or furuncle formation or ascending lymphangitis are more commonly present in these infections than in plague.

Other important causes of acute lymphadenitis include infectious mononucleosis, cytomegaloviral infection, and toxoplasmosis. These diagnoses can be separated from plague through examination of the blood for the presence of atypical lymphocytes and through appropriate serological tests.

In patients with pharyngitis or cervical lymphadenopathy, the diagnosis of *Str. pyogenes* group A must be excluded, in addition to diphtheria, botulism, viral infections, and gonococcal pharyngitis. A throat culture and serological examination serve to establish these diagnoses.

TABLE 4.4
Epidemiologic and Clinical Features of Plague and Tularemia

	Plague	Tularemia
Persons at risk	Persons living under adverse socioeconomic and hygienic conditions, hunters	Hunters, campers
Geographic distribution in the United States	Focal areas in southwestern United States	Widespread throughout the United States
Seasonal incidence	Summer, fall	All year, dependent on hunting seasons
Animal reservoirs	Squirrels, prairie dogs, chipmunks, marmots, mice, rats	Rabbits, squirrels, woodchucks, muskrats, beavers
Vectors	Fleas	Ticks, deerflies, horseflies
Transmission other than by animals and vectors	Inhalation	Ingestion of water or uncooked meat, inhalation
Portal of entry	Skin, lungs	Skin, conjunctiva, oral or gastrointestinal mucosa, lungs
Incubation period	2 to 8 days	2 to 10 days
Bubo location	Femoral and inguinal most common	Axillary and epitrochlear most common
Skin lesions	Uncommon	Ulcer or pustule usually present
White blood cell count	Elevated with left shift	Usually normal
Bacteria in tissues	Numerous and usually demonstrable by staining or culture of a bubo aspirate	Infrequently seen or cultured
Blood cultures	Commonly positive	Rarely positive
Clinical course	Often fulminant with death	Usually indolent and self-limited
Mortality		
Untreated	50 to 90%	5 to 33%
Treated	5 to 20%	0 to 8%
Complications	Pneumonia, meningitis, shock	Pneumonia, pericarditis, meningitis

In patients with pneumonia who do not have the common bacterial causes, a work-up should be performed not only for tularemia and plague but also for psittacosis, Q fever, mycoplasma infection, tuberculosis, fungal infections, and influenza or other viral infections. Many of these agents will be suggested by the history or can be detected by appropriate cultures, stains, and serologies. Legionnaires' disease may also be a relevant consideration.

Dyspnea and diarrhea occur more frequently in legionnaires' disease than in the other pneumonias. Legionnaires' disease is usually diagnosed by the indirect fluorescent antibody test against the legionnaires' bacterium, *Legionella pneumophila*. However, incorrect diagnoses of legionnaires' disease have been made in patients who later were proved to have plague, tularemia, and leptospirosis, presumably because of cross-reacting antigens.

4.1.13. Mortality

The prognosis of plague in the preantibiotic era was abysmal. In Yersin's first description of plague bacillus in Hong Kong in 1894, he reported that about 95% of patients died. Similarly, in the United States most of the patients died, but the diagnosis was usually established at autopsy, and these reports of very high case–fatality rates may be misleading about the prognosis of all patients with plague. The range that is often quoted is 50–90% mortality. In pneumonic plague the mortality is similarly high, and it was the experience in Madagascar that all patients died unless they received treatment within 20 hr after the onset of symptoms.[18] The case–fatality rate of plague in the United States during the antibiotic era of the 1970s was still 14%. Thus, the presence of fatalities in the setting of acute regional lymphadenitis remains a hallmark of bubonic plague.

4.2. *YERSINIA ENTEROCOLITICA* INFECTION

In the pathogenesis of *Yersinia enterocolitica* infection, the bacteria are presumably ingested and proliferate in the lumen of the bowel and in the lymphoid tissue of the intestines where they cause acute inflammation. Less commonly the bacteria disseminate by way of the blood to the joints or other organs to produce extraintestinal inflammation. The four common clinical syndromes that are caused by *Y. enterocolitica* include (1) acute enteritis with fever and diarrhea, (2) abdominal pain in the right lower quadrant that may mimic acute appendicitis, (3) arthritis, and (4) erythema nodosum.[27–45] In any one patient one or more of these syndromes may appear, or there may be one of the rarer forms of septicemia, iritis, myocarditis, abscesses of the liver and spleen, osteomyelitis, and meningitis. Thus, *Y. enterocolitica* infections, even more so than plague infection, are a challenge and fascination for the diagnostician in medicine. The surgeon, nearly as often as the internist, sees patients with these infections because of the severe abdominal pain that frequently is localized in the right lower quadrant and results in unnecessary laparotomies for appendectomy.

Several organ systems may be involved by *Y. enterocolitica* infection, so other diseases are frequently mimicked. The pathogenesis of the arthritis and erythema nodosum, in most cases, appears to be delayed immunological sequellae of the original intestinal infection. The greater likelihood that patients with the genotype HLA-B27 will develop arthritis during an infection with *Y. enterocolitica* suggests that this organism produces some of its clinical manifestation through the immune responses of each patient to the microbial antigens.[31]

4.2.1. Acute Enteritis

This is the most common clinical form in most of the larger series of reported cases (Table 4.5) and typically manifests as fever and diarrhea. Young children and infants are predominantly affected, and the disease is usually mild and self-limited.[46,47] The character of the diarrhea varies from watery to mucoid and even grossly bloody stools. Abdominal pain and vom-

TABLE 4.5
Frequency of Clinical Syndromes Caused by *Yersinia enterocolitica*

	Numbers of cases (percent)			
Clinical report	Enteritis with diarrhea and fever	Abdominal pain or appendicitislike syndrome	Arthritis or arthralgia	Erythema nodosum
Nilehn *et al.*[94] (31 cases)	24 (77)	12 (39)	6 (19)	10 (32)
Nilehn and Sjostrom[30] (150 cases)[a]	58 (39)	83 (55)	"Occasional"	17 (11)
Ahvonen[29] (304 cases)	198 (65)	36 (12)	101 (33)	97 (32)
Leino and Kalliomaki[56] (60 cases)[b]	27 (45)	20 (33)	33 (55)	11 (18)
Black *et al.*[50] (38 cases)	18 (47)	22 (58)	2 (5)	0 (0)

[a] These 150 cases include the 31 previously reported.
[b] Fifty-six of these cases were caused by *Y. enterocolitica*, four by *Y. pseudotuberculosis*.

iting frequently accompany the diarrhea. Polymorphonuclear leukocytes have been found in stools of patients, indicating that it is an inflammatory, invasive form of diarrhea. Accordingly, the white blood cell count is usually elevated with an increased proportion of young forms. Thus, the clinical picture of *Y. enterocolitica* enteritis initially resembles that of *Shigella, Salmonella,* or amebic diarrhea. The duration of illness is usually 2 to 3 weeks, but occasionally longer courses have suggested the diagnosis of chronic inflammatory bowel disease. This protracted course of the diarrhea can assist the clinician to distinguish yersiniosis from other acute diarrheal diseases which usually run a shorter course.

The pathology of the small bowel in the enteritis syndrome has rarely been studied because surgery and autopsies are not usually performed. In Japan, Zen-Yoji and Maruyama described two fatal cases of *Y. enterocolitica* infection, in which the ileocecal region of the small bowel showed extensive hemorrhagic necrosis.[(48)] In the appendicitislike syndrome the terminal ileum is often acutely inflamed, suggesting that the enteritis is predominantly an ileitis. The large intestine also was involved in two fatal cases in the United States reported by Gutman *et al.*[(49)] In one of these cases a hemicolectomy was performed because of extensive bleeding. The terminal ileum, ascending colon, and transverse colon showed inflammation of the mucosa and submucosa with ulcerations and abscesses.

4.2.2. Abdominal Pain and Appendicitislike Syndrome

Many patients with *Y. enterocolitica* infection do not develop diarrhea but have a clinical picture dominated by abdominal pain and fever. Whereas infants and other children less than 5 years predominantly develop gastroenteritis, older children and adults more often develop this syndrome of abdominal pain. Typically the pain and abdominal tenderness are most severe in the right lower quadrant, giving rise to the suspected diagnosis of appendicitis. When there is terminal ileitis caused by *Y. enterocolitica,* the correct diagnosis is usually revealed at laparotomy by a normal appendix with an inflamed ileum. In other patients with right lower quadrant tenderness, there may be only mesenteric lymphadenitis. Here, the clinician may suspect *Y. enterocolitica* infection, rather than appendicitis, after demonstrating that the area of maximum tenderness shifts when the patient is moved from side to side.[(35)] This clinical picture may resemble typhoid fever. Helpful distinguishing features are that *Y. enterocolitica* infection has a more abrupt onset dominated by abdominal pain and that the white blood cell count is usually elevated with an increased proportion of young forms. In the patients reported by Black *et al.*,[(50)] the mean white blood cell count was 12,115/mm^3.

In Belgium, Vantrappen *et al.*[(51,52)] have carried out radiographic, endoscopic, and histologic studies that have helped to define the physiopathology of *Yersinia* enteritis. In 24 patients examined by X-ray contrast methods, abnormalities of the ileum were detected in 21 cases. The most frequent sign was thickening of the mucosal folds or a nodular mucosal pattern. Mucosal ulcerations were present in about half of the cases. The ulcers were either solitary or multiple and included both aphthoid ulcers like those seen in Crohn's disease, which are elevated and therefore displace the contrast material, and longitudinal ulcers of 2 cm or more in length. Other findings were thickening of the ileal wall, dilatation of the lumen, hypercontractility, and lacunar images caused by the pressure of adjacent enlarged mesenteric lymph nodes. During the course of *Yersinia* infection, the earliest changes were thickening of the mucosal folds and the nodular pattern. Late in the course and after more than a month during convalescence, there may persist some small filling defects 1 to 2 mm in diameter in the mucosa. In most cases, complete healing was observed after recovery. Barium enemas of the colon showed less striking changes, but some patients showed mucosal ulcerations. Endoscopic examination of the colon showed that half of the patients were entirely normal. In other patients, the mucosa was erythematous, edematous, and friable. Small ulcerations resembling aphthoid ulcers of Crohn's disease were seen in some patients. These ulcers were shallow, round, yellow-white, and 1 to 2 mm in diameter. The yellow-white covering could be removed, leaving sharply demarcated ulcers with a red base. The mucosa between the ulcers appeared normal. In contrast to those of Crohn's disease, the ulcers were nearly uniform in size. Biopsies of these colonic ulcers revealed an inflammatory infiltrate of the lamina propria consisting of predominantly polymorphonuclear leukocytes. The epithelial cell layer showed necrosis, and only the superficial third of the crypts were necrotic in these superficial ulcers. Lymphoid cell aggregations were present in these areas of ulceration. In some cases, the mucosal surface was covered by a "pseudomembrane" or mucoid debris.

The pathology of the appendicitislike syndrome has been amply described because laparotomies have been frequently performed for suspected appendicitis. In the largest clinical series reported to date, Ahvonen reported in 1972 on 304 cases of *Y. enterocolitica* infection in Finland.[(29)] Thirty-six of these patients underwent laparotomy. In 28 cases the appendix was entirely normal and in eight the appendix was mildly inflamed, showing focal ulceration of the appendical mucosa; in 34 of the operated patients the mesenteric lymph nodes were enlarged and the histology of the nodes showed a proliferation of pyroninophilic cells.

In Sweden, Nilehn, and Sjostrom examined 581 consecutive patients who underwent appendectomy during a 1-year period for *Y. enterocolitica* infection.[(30)] The bacterium was isolated from 22 (3.8%) of all patients. When the postoperative diagnoses were established, *Y. enterocolitica* was more frequently isolated from patients with terminal ileitis (80% of the cases) and mesenteric lymphadenitis (13% of the cases) than from patients with verified acute appendicitis (only 0.6% of the cases). Furthermore, *Y. enterocolitica* was more frequently isolated in patients initially suspected of having appendicitis but not operated on (5.6% of patients) than in the group operated on. In 974 control patients without abdominal pain, *Y. enterocolitica* was isolated from only one case. These results suggested that *Y. enterocolitica* is rarely a cause of acute appendicitis, but is a relatively common cause of ileitis and mesenteric lymphadenitis.

In a similar prospective study of 244 patients in Denmark with acute abdominal pain, Jepsen *et al.*[(53)] diagnosed *Y. enterocolitica* infection in 22 patients (9%), of which 15 went to surgery. Table 4.6 shows that the common surgical findings were a mildly inflamed appendix, a normal appendix with inflamed mesenteric lymph nodes, and severe appendicitis with ulceration or suppuration. When these findings were compared to a control group of operated patients without *Yersinia* infection, the control group more often had the findings of severe typical appendicitis. However, the operative findings overlapped in the two groups.

In the United States, Black *et al.*[(50)] reported the operative findings in 16 children with *Y. enterocolitica* appendicitislike syndrome. The most common finding was enlarged mesenteric lymph nodes (10 cases); also frequent were an inflamed terminal ileum (four cases) and an erythematous appendix (four cases). Histological examinations of these 16 appendices showed that eight were normal, five showed suppuration, and three showed lymphoid hyperplasia. In Japan, Fukushima *et al.*[(54)] have described cases of appendicitis caused by *Y. enterocolitica*. The appendices showed inflammation, congestion, and edema.

TABLE 4.6
Frequency of Pathological Changes in the Appendices of 15 Patients with *Yersinia* Infection Who Underwent Appendectomy Compared to 106 Patients without *Yersinia* Infection[a]

	Yersinia infection (15 patients)	Without *Yersinia* infection (106 patients)
Normal appendix and mesenteric lymph nodes	0 (0%)	17 (17%)
Normal appendix with inflamed mesenteric lymph nodes	4 (27%)	7 (6%)
Mild inflammation of appendix (catarrhal)	8 (53%)	28 (26%)
Severe inflammation of appendix (ulceration, suppuration, or perforation)	3[b] (20%)	54 (51%)

[a] Adapted from Jepsen *et al.*[53] with permission of author and publisher.
[b] There were no perforated appendices in the *Yersinia* infections.

Although the pathological descriptions of patients in the several available sources have varied according to severity and location of inflammation in the intestine, some of the common features have been elucidated by Bradford *et al.*[55] As in *Y. pestis* infection, there is hyperplasia and acute inflammation of lymphoid tissue in which the causative bacteria are proliferating and producing hemorrhage and necrosis. The intestinal pathology of *Y. enterocolitica* resembles grossly that of typhoid fever with prominent lymphoid follicles producing ulceration of the overlying intestinal mucosa. Whereas the cellular response in *Salmonella* is predominantly mononuclear, it is mainly polymorphonuclear in *Yersinia* enteritis. The lymphoid tissue that characteristically is hypertrophied includes the Peyer's patches of the ileum, the submucosal lymphoid follicles of the appendix, and the mesenteric lymph nodes. Bradford *et al.* noted that ulcerations of the intestinal mucosa were most prominent at sites of lymphoid tissue. Some sections of bowel showed lymphoid tissue, affected by necrosis and polymorphonuclear infiltration, extending through the muscularis layer to the overlying ulcerated mucosa.[55] In the majority of cases of *Y. enterocolitica* enteritis, which are nonfatal, the inflammatory process is confined to the terminal ileum or mesenteric lymph nodes, whereas the colon has been affected in some fatal cases that have produced grossly bloody diarrhea.[49]

4.2.3. Arthritis

The most common extraintestinal form of *Y. enterocolitica* infection, in some of the series shown in Table 4.5, is arthritis. In Finland, arthritis appears to be relatively more common, occurring in about a third to a half of the patients described by Ahvonen[(29)] and Leino and Kalliomaki,[(56)] but many of the case reports from elsewhere, including the United States, confirm that arthritis is commonly associated with *Yersinia* infection. Adults are predominantly affected by arthritis, whereas the gastroenteritis and appendicitislike syndromes occur predominantly in children.

The largest clinical experiences with *Yersinia* arthritis have been reported by Ahvonen and colleagues.[(33)] They reported a series of 101 patients, of whom 88 developed arthritis during or soon after febrile gastroenteritis or appendicitislike illness. The majority of patients (89) experienced polyarthritis, whereas only 12 patients had monarthritis. The order of frequency of the affected joints were knees, ankles, toes and tarsal joints, fingers, wrists, elbows, and sternoclavicular and sacroiliac joints. Typically, the joints were involved one after another, in a migratory manner, and the average maximum number of 2.9 joints per patient was usually affected within 1 week. Symptoms lasted from 1 to 3 months in most cases. The joints were tender and frequently had effusions. Synovial fluid obtained from 32 cases showed leukocyte counts from 400 to 63,000/mm^3 with 59 to 95% polymorphonuclear leukocytes. Cultures of synovial fluid were sterile, and glucose concentrations were normal. Tests for rheumatoid factors were usually negative, but six cases showed positive latex tests and two had elevated titers of the Waaler–Rose test. Subsequent to their initial report, these Finnish workers have demonstrated a predilection of persons with the HLA-B27 antigen to develop arthritis as a complication of *Yersinia* infection.[(31)] They found the HLA-B27 antigen in 9 of 11 females and all of 11 males examined with *Yersinia* arthritis. Reiter's syndrome, including conjunctivitis urethritis, and arthritis, has also been reported in individuals with HLA-B27 antigen following a *Yersinia* infection.[(57)]

This clinical picture of *Yersinia* arthritis is a "reactive" arthritis, rather than a septic arthritis, and resembles the arthritis associated with *Shigella, Salmonella, Brucella,* and gonococcal infections, as well as the arthritis of acute rheumatic fever. Thus, the evaluation of patients with arthritis associated with enteric disease requires careful attention to stool cultures and serological testing.

In addition to this typical picture of nonseptic reactive arthritis, *Y. enterocolitica* can also produce septic arthritis. Two cases are recorded in the American literature.[41] Both were older men who did not have a preceding intestinal syndrome but had positive blood cultures for *Y. enterocolitica* in addition to positive cultures of synovial fluid.

4.2.4. Erythema Nodosum

With the exception of the American series of Black *et al.*,[50] all of the larger reports of *Y. enterocolitica* infection show a strong association with erythema nodosum. Ahvonen[29] reported 106 cases, in which females outnumbered males 92 to 14, whereas in the entire group of infected patients there was a female/male ratio of about 2 to 1. This female prevalence of erythema nodosum was also observed by Leino and Kalliomaki who reported 10 females and one male with this clinical sign.[56] The patients showed the typical tender nodules on the anterior aspect of legs and some patients also had nodules on their arms. Some patients with erythema nodosum gave histories of having had it on previous occasions, suggesting that the *Yersinia* infection provokes in a nonspecific manner some underlying tendency to develop this acute inflammatory reaction.

4.2.5. Septicemia and Generalized Infections

The majority of patients with *Yersinia* infections with intestinal manifestations have negative blood cultures and no evidence for disseminated infection. Even the common extraintestinal complications of arthritis and erythema nodosum appear to be reactions to the enteritic infection, rather than due to the presence of bacteria at extraintestinal sites. Rarely, however, the infection cannot be contained in the gut-associated lymphoid tissue and appears in the blood. Mollaret[58] drew attention to the striking association of disseminated *Y. enterocolitica* with liver cirrhosis, diabetes, and the hematological conditions thalassemia, aplastic anemia, and leukemia. Rabson *et al.*[59] reported 13 cases of generalized infection in South Africa. Nine of these patients had cirrhosis, four of whom showed signs of hemochromatosis from iron overload due to drinking alcoholic beverages that contain excessive ionized iron. Other case reports of septicemic *Yersinia* infections have been reported in patients, some of whom had thalassemia and hemochromatosis.[60–62] These underlying diseases point to the reticuloendothelial system of the liver as the essential defense against dissemination of infection in normal individuals. Whether the liver is damaged by cirrhosis or the Kupffer cells are saturated by hemolyzing red cells in hemoglobinopathies, it can be assumed that the usually low-grade portal venous bacteremia gains greater access to the systemic circulation to result in disseminated infection. Some of the patients with thalassemia that developed disseminated infection had been previously splenectomized,[60,63] and the absence of the splenic reticuloendothelial and antibody-forming tissues may have further predisposed these patients to systemic infection. Still another mechanism that has been proposed for disseminated infection is the effect of iron overload in hemochromatosis and hemolytic conditions. This suggestion is based on the observation that iron may enhance the virulence of the bacteria.[59]

In the patients reported by Rabson *et al.*[59,64] there were two clinical patterns. The acute septicemic form consisted of fever, abdominal pain, diarrhea, enlarged liver, and leukocytosis. Most had jaundice. The differential diagnosis included malaria and typhoid fever. In the second form, the subacute localizing form, the clinical presentation did not include diarrhea and vomiting. Spleens were usually palpable, and these patients had large abscesses of the liver and spleen. The clinical diagnosis was often amebic hepatitis before culture results showed the correct diagnosis. The mortality rate in this report of generalized *Yersinia* infection was 6 of 13 patients. All six deaths had the subacute localizing form of the disease. Liver abscess due to *Y. enterocolitica* was described by Viteri *et al.*[65] in the United States. This patient did not have diarrhea but was a diabetic who had undergone oral surgery with antibiotic coverage 2 weeks before his illness.

4.2.6. Miscellaneous Clinical Forms

A large variety of rare clinical forms of *Y. enterocolitica* infection have been observed. This organism can produce acute pharyngitis and tonsillitis, which were prominent features of the epidemic described by Gutman *et al.*[49] Cervical lymphadenitis with or without pharyngitis may be caused by *Y. enterocolitica;* a case in a child recently reported by Jaffe and Smith[66] consisted of anterior cervical adenitis with an overlying draining ulcer.

Other forms include osteomyelitis, meningitis, myocarditis, iritis, glomerulonephritis, and pulmonary infections.[67] The first two represent rare forms of metastatic localization of infection. Osteomyelitis has occurred in some patients with thalassemia.[63,68] Perhaps in these patients, as in the *Salmonella* osteomyelitis of sickle cell disease, bony infarcts that occur as a result of the hemoglobinopathy provide a good nidus for the infection during bacteremia.

Meningitis caused by *Y. enterocolitica* was reported from the United States by Challa and Marx.[69] This patient was an alcoholic with cirrhosis and died with meningitis. The unusual serotype O:18 was cultured from the brain at autopsy, which showed necrosis in the globus pallidus and ependyma, meningeal infiltration with lymphocytes and plasma cells, perivascular inflammation, and fibrin thrombi in blood vessels.

Myocarditis as a complication of *Yersinia* infection was stressed by Ahvonen *et al.*[32] who noted that 5 of 25 patients with *Y. enterocolitica* arthritis showed transient prolonged PR intervals or T-wave inversions. Because of fever, arthritis, and myocarditis the diagnosis of rheumatic fever was considered in these patients, who had no evidence of antecedent streptococcal infection. This report shows the need to consider *Yersinia* infection in the symptom complex that suggests rheumatic fever. Leino and Kalliomaki[56] also observed myocarditis in 4 of 60 patients with *Yersinia* infection. Electrocardiograms showed ST-segment elevation and T-wave inversions.

A further analogy with poststreptococcal syndromes has been suggested by a report of glomerulonephritis, which followed by 2 weeks an episode of *Yersinia* gastroenteritis and arthritis. This patient had hematuria and proteinuria, and the renal biopsy showed glomerular deposits of immunoglobulin and complement.[70]

Lung infections caused by *Y. enterocolitica* are rare, but several cases have been reported. The most common pulmonary syndrome is pulmonary infiltrates with septicemia, in which the organism is isolated from blood and sputum. Here the presumed pathogenesis is intestinal infection followed by dissemination of bacteria to the lung via the blood.[71] Other syndromes include hilar adenopathy[72] and lung abscess with cavitation. In one case, lung abscesses developed in a patient with a colonic carcinoma, suggesting that the colon was the portal of entry for *Y. enterocolitica.*[73]

4.3. *YERSINIA PSEUDOTUBERCULOSIS* INFECTION

This organism is a well-recognized cause of acute mesenteric lymphadenitis in Europe. In Germany in 1958 Knapp summarized information on 117 cases, which had been diagnosed by isolation of the bacterium from inflamed lymph nodes in 13 cases and from the blood in two cases, and had been serologically diagnosed by agglutinin titers in the remaining patients.[74] The major pathological feature of these cases was mesenteric lymphadenitis which consisted of enlarged follicles and abscesses; occasionally, the same patients had inflammatory reactions in the terminal ileum, cecum, or appendix. Ahvonen in 1972 described features of 30 cases from Finland, which were serologically diagnosed in 27 cases and by isolation of *Yersinia pseudotuberculosis* from appendices of two cases and stool of one case.[29] Twenty-seven had fever, 20 had abdominal pain, and seven had diarrhea. Appendectomies were performed in 10 patients, which had operative findings of enlarged mesenteric lymph nodes in nine cases. None had ileitis or appendicitis. Associated clinical findings included erythema nodosum in 14 patients and polyarthritis in three patients.

In the second largest clinical series of *Y. pseudotuberculosis* to date, El-Maraghi and Mair[75] reported in 1979 findings of surgical pathology in 70 cases from England. The preoperative diagnosis was appendicitis in all cases except one in whom it was mesenteric adenitis. The operative findings included mesenteric lymphadenopathy involving ileocecal nodes in 69 cases, terminal ileitis in 13 cases, and acute appendicitis in two cases. They described the characteristic pathological changes in the mesenteric lymph nodes as consisting of four stages: (1) lymphoid hyperplasia, (2) histiocytic cell hyperplasia, (3) epithelioid granulomatous changes, and (4) central coagulative necrosis of the granulomas. Langhan's giant cells, suggestive of tuberculosis, were seen in only one case. The histology of the ileum was similar to that of the lymph nodes, consisting of lymphoid tissue hyperplasia, necrotizing granulomas, panmural inflammation, and mucosal ulceration.

In these larger series of patients and other case reports, the clinical picture and pathology of *Y. pseudotuberculosis* infection closely resembles that of *Y. enterocolitica* infection. There are, however, some suggestions of differences between these infections (Table 4.7). The lower incidence of diarrhea and of positive stool cultures in *Y. pseudotuberculosis* infection may reflect a less rapid proliferation of this organism in the bowel lumen. Accordingly, *Y. pseudotuberculosis* produces pathology that is dominated by mesenteric lymphadenitis with enteritis being less common and generally milder than that of *Y. enterocolitica*. Existing clinical descriptions suggest that the extraintestinal effects of arthritis and erythema nodosum are less common in *Y. pseudotuberculosis* than in *Y. enterocolitica,* but this may be merely the result

TABLE 4.7
Contrasting of Clinical and Pathological Features of Infections Caused by *Yersinia enterocolitica* and *Yersinia pseudotuberculosis*

	Y. enterocolitica	*Y. pseudotuberculosis*
Clinical	Diarrhea common	Diarrhea rare
Stool cultures	Usually positive	Usually negative
Intestinal pathology	Terminal ileitis common; appendix usually normal but occasionally inflamed with microabscesses and necrosis	Ileum usually normal; appendix may show mild inflammation
Mesenteric lymph nodes	Inflamed with necrosis and histiocytic inflammatory response	Inflamed with reticular cell proliferation and granulocytic cell response

of fewer total cases of the former infection having been recognized and carefully observed. Several other reports have described smaller numbers of cases.[76–79]

In the normal host, *Y. pseudotuberculosis* is a self-limited and relatively mild disease. It runs its course in 1–2 weeks and does not seem to be affected by antibiotic treatment. The greatest hazard that these patients face is the possibility of undergoing laparotomy for suspected appendicitis.

In the United States, *Y. pseudotuberculosis* mesenteric lymphadenitis has been infrequently diagnosed. In 1971 Hubbert *et al.*[76] reported that only five cases had been recorded in medical literature, and they added two new ones. Most of these have occurred in the western United States.

In addition to the typical syndrome of mesenteric lymphadenitis, *Y. pseudotuberculosis* can produce septicemia that is frequently fatal. In 1971, there was a flurry of clinical articles describing this syndrome.[80–82] At that time 21 cases of *Y. pseudotuberculosis* sepsis were identified in the world's literature, of whom 10 had underlying cirrhosis due to alcoholism or hemochromatosis; 17 of the patients died. These reports added five cases of sepsis from the United States; two had hemochromatosis, two had polycythemia vera (of whom one also had myeloid metaplasia and one had liver fibrosis), and one was apparently healthy. Two of these five patients died. Two patients in Norway were reported with septicemia caused by *Y. pseudotuberculosis*.[83,84] Both of these patients had underlying liver disease; one had chronic active hepatitis treated with corticosteroids and azathioprine and one had amyloidosis. Another patient reported from Korea with *Y. pseudotuberculosis* sepsis had cirrhosis.[85] The predisposition of patients with cirrhosis and other liver diseases to develop the severe form of disseminated *Y. pseudotuberculosis* infection suggests that, as in *Y. enterocolitica* infection, the normal liver plays a dominant role in protecting patients with localized intestinal infections from progressing to systemic sepsis.

REFERENCES

1. F. M. Burkle, Plague as seen in South Vietnamese children: A chronicle of observations and treatment under adverse conditions, *Clin. Pediatr.* **12:**291–298 (1973).
2. T. Butler, A clinical study of bubonic plague: Observation of the 1970 Vietnam epidemic with emphasis on coagulation studies, skin histology, and electrocardiograms, *Am. J. Med.* **53:**268–276 (1972).
3. N. N. Thuat and N. D. Tiep, Clinical considerations and therapeutics in 500 confirmed plague patients in Cho-Quan Hospital, Symposium on Plague, Saigon, October 1970.
4. L. F. Barker, On the clinical aspects of plague, *Am. J. Med. Sci.* **122:**377–395 (1901).
5. J. R. Cantey, Plague in Vietnam: Clinical observations and treatment with kanamycin, *Arch. Intern. Med.* **133:**280–283 (1974).
6. F. G. Conrad, F. R. LeCocq, and R. Krain, A recent epidemic of plague in Vietnam, *Arch. Intern. Med.* **122:**193–198 (1968).
7. L. J. Legters, A. J. Cottingham, and D. H. Hunter, Clinical and epidemiologic notes on a defined outbreak of plague in Vietnam, *Am. J. Trop. Med. Hyg.* **19:**639–652 (1970).
8. C. G. Reiley and E. D. Kates, The clinical spectrum of plague in Vietnam, *Arch. Intern. Med.* **126:**990–994 (1970).
9. W. P. Reed, D. L. Palmer, R. C. Williams, and A. L. Kisch, Bubonic plague in the Southwestern United States, *Medicine* **49:**465–486 (1970).
10. S. Flexner, The pathology of bubonic plague, *Am. J. Med. Sci.* **122:**396–416 (1901).
11. T. L. Stahly and J. D. Shoop, Plague and gallium scan: Case report, *J. Nucl. Med.* **16:**1031–1032 (1975).
12. M. E. White, R. D. Rosenbaum, T. M. Canfield, and J. D. Poland, Plague in a neonate, *Am. J. Dis. Child.* **135:**418–419 (1981).
13. B. Velimirovic, Personal communication, color photographs from papers by J. Stockard and B. J. Mulholland delivered at Teheran Congress of Tropical Medicine and Malaria, 1968.
14. T. Butler, Plague and tularemia, *Pediatr. Clin. North Am.* **26:**355–360 (1979).
15. T. Butler, J. Levin, D. Q. Cu, and R. I. Walker, Bubonic plague: Detection of endotoxemia with the limulus test, *Ann. Intern. Med.* **79:**642–646 (1973).
16. T. Butler, W. R. Bell, N. N. Linh, N. D. Tiep, and K. Arnold, *Yersinia pestis* infection in Vietnam I. Clinical and hematologic aspects, *J. Infect. Dis.* **129**(Suppl)**:**S78–S84 (1974).
17. T. Butler, J. Levin, N. N. Linh, D. M. Chau, M. Adickman, and K. Arnold, *Yersinia pestis* infection in Vietnam II. Quantitative blood cultures and detection of endotoxin in the cerebrospinal fluid of patients with meningitis, *J. Infect. Dis.* **133:**493–499 (1976).
18. F. R. McCrumb, S. Mercier, J. Robic, M. Bouillat, J. E. Smadel, T. E. Woodward, and K. Goodner, Chloramphenicol and terramycin in the treatment of pneumonic plague, *Am. J. Med.* **41:**284–293 (1953).

19. P. Trong, T. Q. Nhu, and J. D. Marshall, A mixed pneumonic bubonic plague outbreak in Vietnam, *Milit. Med.* **132:**93–97 (1967).
20. R. J. Cohen and J. L. Stockard, Pneumonic plague in an untreated plague-vaccinated individual, *J. Am. Med. Assoc.* **202:**217–218 (1967).
21. C. F. von Reyn, N. S. Weber, B. Tempest, A. M. Barnes, J. D. Poland, J. M. Boyce, and V. Zalma, Epidemiologic and clinical features of an outbreak of bubonic plague in New Mexico, *J. Infect. Dis.* **136:**489–494 (1977).
22. J. D. Marshall, D. V. Quy, and F. L. Gibson, Asymptomatic pharyngeal plague infection in Vietnam, *Am. J. Trop. Med. Hyg.* **16:**175–177 (1967).
23. R. L. Washington, R. M. Barkin, and J. R. Hillman, Septicemic plague that mimics Reye's syndrome, *Am. J. Dis. Child.* **133:**434–435 (1979).
24. J. Schwade and J. P. Sanford, Hepatic granuloma due to benign plague imported from Vietnam: Case report, *Milit. Med.* **139:**554–556 (1974).
25. M. J. Finegold, Pathogenesis of plague: A review of plague deaths in the United States during the last decade, *Am. J. Med.* **45:**549–554 (1968).
26. V. R. Sites, J. D. Poland, and B. W. Hudson, Bubonic plague misdiagnosed as tularemia, *J. Am. Med. Assoc.* **222:**1642–1643 (1972).
27. S. Winblad, B. Nilehn, and M. Jonsson, Two further cases, bacteriologically verified, of human infection with *Pasteurella X* (Syn. *Yersinia enterocolitica*), *Acta Pathol. Microbiol. Scand.* **67:**537–541 (1966).
28. S. Winblad, B. Nilehn, and N. H. Sternby, *Yersinia enterocolitica (Pasteurella X)* in human enteric infections, *Br. Med. J.* **2:**1363–1366 (1966).
29. P. Ahvonen, Human yersiniosis in Finland II. Clinical features. *Ann. Clin. Res.* **4:**39–48 (1972).
30. B. Nilehn and B. Sjostrom, Studies on *Yersinia enterocolitica:* Occurrence in various groups of acute abdominal disease, *Acta Pathol. Microbiol. Scand.* **71:**612–628 (1967).
31. K. Aho, P. Ahvonen, A. Lassus, K. Sievers, and A. Tiilikainen, HL-A antigen and reactive arthritis, *Lancet* **2:**157 (1973).
32. P. Ahvonen, L. Hiisi-Brummer, and K. Aho, Electrocardiographic abnormalities and arthritis in patients with *Yersinia enterocolitica* infection, *Ann. Clin. Res.* **3:**69–75 (1971).
33. P. Ahvonen, K. Sievers, and K. Aho, Arthritis associated with *Yersinia enterocolitica* infection, *Acta Rheumatol. Scand.* **15:**232–253 (1969).
34. N. E. Baldock and M. D. Catterall, Erythema nodosum from *Yersinia enterocolitica, Br. J. Dermatol.* **93:**719–720 (1975).
35. R. J. Blattner, Acute mesenteric lymphadenitis, *J. Pediatr.* **74:**479–481 (1969).
36. E. C. Bonard, Yersinoses, *Schweiz. Med. Wochenschr.* **106:**65–70 (1976).
37. H. Braunstein, E. B. Tucker, and B. C. Gibson, Mesenteric lymphadenitis due to *Yersinia enterocolitica:* Report of a case, *Am. J. Clin. Pathol.* **55:**506–510 (1971).
38. M. J. Brodie, P. A. Boot, and R. W. A. Girdwood, Severe *Yersinia pseudotuberculosis* infection diagnosed at laparoscopy, *Br. Med. J.* **3:**88 (1973).
39. D. Y. Bulgen, B. L. Hazleman, and R. E. Warren, Arthritis and neuralgic amyotrophy due to *Yersinia enterocolitica, Br. Med. J.* **1:**1250 (1979).
40. N. V. Doraiswamy, A. B. M. Currie, J. Gray, and C. Lynton-Moll, Terminal ileitis: *Yersinia enterocolitica* isolated from faeces, *Br. Med. J.* **2:**23–25 (1977).
41. J. C. Jacobs, *Yersinia enterocolitica* arthritis, *Pediatr.* **55:**236–238 (1975).
42. E. Jansson, G. R. Wallgren, and P. Ahvonen, *Yersinia enterocolitica* as a cause of acute mesenteric lymphadenitis, *Acta Pediatr. Scand.* **57:**448–450 (1968).
43. N. Mygind and H. Thulin, *Yersinia enterocolitica:* A new cause of erythema nodosum, *Br. J. Derm.* **82:**351–354 (1970).

44. B. C. Schieven and C. Randall, Enteritis due to *Yersinia enterocolitica, J. Pediatr.* **84:**402–404 (1974).
45. J. T. Scott and N. S. Mair, *Yersinia* arthritis, *Br. Med. J.* **1:**1251 (1979).
46. S. Kohl, J. A. Jacobson, and A. Nahmias, *Yersinia enterocolitica* infections in children, *J. Pediatr.* **89:**77–79 (1976).
47. W. J. Rodriguez, G. Controni, G. J. Cohen, B. Florence, W. N. Khan, and S. Ross, *Yersinia enterocolitica* enteritis in children, *J. Am. Med. Assoc.* **242:**1978–1980 (1980).
48. H. Zen-Yoji and T. Maruyama, The first successful isolations and identification of *Yersinia enterocolitica* from human cases in Japan, *Jpn. J. Microbiol.* **16:**493–500 (1972).
49. L. T. Gutman, E. A. Otteson, T. J. Quan, P. S. Noce, and S. L. Katz, An interfamilial outbreak of *Yersinia enterocolitica* enteritis, *N. Engl. J. Med.* **288:**1372–1377 (1972).
50. R. E. Black, R. J. Jackson, T. Tsai, M. Medvesky, M. Shayegani, J. C. Feeley, K. I. E. MacLeod, and A. M. Wakelee, Epidemic *Yersinia enterocolitica* infection due to contaminated chocolate milk, *N. Engl. J. Med.* **298:**76–79 (1978).
51. G. Vantrappen, H. O. Agg, E. Ponette, K. Geboes, and P. Bertrand, *Yersinia* enteritis and enterocolitis: Gastroenterological aspects, *Gastroenterology* **72:**220–227 (1977).
52. G. Vantrappen, H. O. Agg, K. Geboes, and E. Ponette, *Yersinia* enteritis, *Med. Clin. North Am.* **66:**639–653 (1982).
53. O. B. Jepsen, B. Korner, K. B. Lauritsen, A-B. Hancke, L. Anderson, and S. Henrichsen, *Yersinia enterocolitica* infection in patients with acute surgical abdominal disease: A prospective study, *Scand. J. Infect. Dis.* **8:**189–194 (1976).
54. H. Fukushima, Y. Ito, K. Saito, K. Kuroda, J. Inoue, M. Tsubokura, and K. Otsuki, Intrafamilial cases of *Yersinia enterocolitica* appendicitis, *Microbiol. Immunol.* **25:**71–73 (1981).
55. W. D. Bradford, P. S. Noce, and L. T. Gutman, Pathologic features of enteric infection with *Yersinia enterocolitica, Arch. Pathol.* **98:**17–22 (1974).
56. R. Leino and J. L. Kalliomaki, Yersiniosis as an internal disease, *Ann. Intern. Med.* **81:**458–461 (1974).
57. J. H. Solem and J. Lassen, Reiter's disease following *Yersinia enterocolitica* infection, *Scand. J. Infect. Dis.* **3:**83–85 (1971).
58. H. H. Mollaret, L'infection humaine à *Yersinia enterocolitica* en 1970 à la lumière de 642 cas récents, *Pathol. Biol.* **19:**189–205 (1971).
59. A. R. Rabson, A. F. Hallett, and H. J. Koornhof, Generalized *Yersinia enterocolitica* infection, *J. Infect. Dis.* **131:**447–451 (1975).
60. J. P. Butzler, M. Alexander, A. Segers, N. Cremer, and D. Blum, Enteritis, abscess, and septicemia due to *Yersinia enterocolitica* in a child with thalassemia, *J. Pediatr.* **93:**619–621 (1978).
61. V. Reinicke and B. Korner, Fulminant septicemia caused by *Yersinia enterocolitica, Scand. J. Infect. Dis.* **9:**249–251 (1977).
62. T. J. Spira and S. A. Kabnis, *Yersinia enterocolitica* septicemia with septic arthritis, *Arch. Intern. Med.* **136:**1305–1308 (1976).
63. M. C. Thirumoorthi and A. S. Dajani, *Yersinia enterocolitica* osteomyelitis in a child, *Am. J. Dis. Child.* **132:**578–582 (1978).
64. A. R. Rabson, H. J. Koornhof, J. Notman, and W. G. Maxwell, Hepatosplenic abscesses due to *Yersinia enterocolitica, Br. Med. J.* **30:**341 (1972).
65. A. L. Viteri, P. H. Howard, J. L. May, G. S. Ramesh, and J. W. Roberts, Hepatic abscess due to *Yersinia enterocolitica* without bacteremia, *Gastroenterology* **81:**592–593 (1981).
66. K. M. Jaffe and A. L. Smith, *Yersinia enterocolitica* cervical lymphadenitis. *J. Pediatr.* **97:**937–939 (1980).

67. A. C. Sonnenwirth, Bacteremia with and without meningitis due to *Yersinia enterocolitica, Edwardsiella tarda, Comamonas terrigena,* and *Pseudomonas maltophilia, Am. N.Y. Acad. Sci.* **174:**488–502 (1970).
68. A. S. Hewstone and G. P. Davidson, *Yersinia enterocolitica* with arthritis in a thalassemic child, *Med. J. Aust.* **1:**1035–1938 (1972).
69. V. R. Challa and R. S. Marx, Pathology of *Yersinia enterocolitica* meningitis, *J. Neurol. Neurosurg. Psychiatry* **43:**455–457 (1980).
70. J. Forsstrom, M. Viander, A. Lehtonen, and T. Ekfors, *Yersinia enterocolitica* infection complicated by glomerulonephritis, *Scand. J. Infect. Dis.* **9:**253–256 (1977).
71. D. Portnoy and L. A. Martinez, *Yersinia enterocolitica* septicemia with pneumonia, *Can. Med. Assoc. J.* **120:**61–62 (1979).
72. E. Sairanen, Hilar adenopathy with *Yersinia* infection, *Ann. Intern. Med.* **80:**673–674 (1974).
73. R. D. Bigler, R. R. Atkins, and E. J. Wing, *Yersinia enterocolitica* lung infection, *Arch. Intern. Med.* **141:**1529–1530 (1981).
74. W. Knapp, Mesenteric adenitis due to *Pasteurella pseudotuberculosis* in young people, *N. Engl. J. Med.* **259:**776–778 (1958).
75. N. R. H. El-Maraghi and N. S. Mair, The histopathology of enteric infection with *Yersinia pseudotuberculosis, Am. J. Clin. Pathol.* **71:**631–639 (1979).
76. W. T. Hubbert, C. W. Petenji, L. A. Glasgow, C. Uyeda, and S. A. Creighton, *Yersinia pseudotuberculosis* infection in the United States, *Am. J. Trop. Med. Hyg.* **20:**679–684 (1971).
77. N. B. Finlayson and B. Fagundes, *Pasteurella pseudotuberculosis* infection: Three cases in the United States, *Am. J. Clin. Pathol.* **55:**24–29 (1971).
78. N. S. Mair, H. J. Mair, E. M. Stirk, and J. G. Corson, Three cases of acute mesenteric lymphadenitis due to *Pasteurella pseudotuberculosis, J. Clin. Pathol.* **13:**432–439 (1960).
79. J. Weber, N. B. Finlayson, and J. B. D. Mark, Mesenteric lymphadenitis and terminal ileitis due to *Yersinia pseudotuberculosis, N. Engl. J. Med.* **283:**172–174 (1970).
80. J. Borowski, M. L. Zaremba, and L. Wasiluk, Fatal septicemia due to *Yersinia pseudotuberculosis, Br. Med. J.* **1:**556 (1971).
81. A. Marlon, L. Gentry, and T. C. Merigan, Septicemia with *Pasteurella pseudotuberculosis, Arch. Intern. Med.* **127:**947–949 (1971).
82. K. M. Yamashiro, R. H. Goldman, D. Harris, and C. T. Uyeda, *Pasteurella pseudotuberculosis:* Acute sepsis with survival, *Arch. Intern. Med.* **128:**605–608 (1971).
83. L. Bevanger, *Yersinia pseudotuberculosis* as the cause of septicaemia in a patient with amyloidosis, *Acta Pathol. Microbiol. Scand. B* **81:**461–462 (1976).
84. T. Gundersen and H. C. Neess, *Yersinia pseudotuberculosis* as the cause of septicaemia in a patient with liver cirrhosis. *Acta Pathol. Microbiol. Scand. B* **89:**61–62 (1981).
85. Y. Chong, Y. C. Kim, S. Y. Lee, and J. K. Kang, *Yersinia pseudotuberculosis* septicemia: Report of a case, *Yonsei Med. J.* **21:**75–79 (1980).
86. K. F. Meyer, C. L. Connor, F. S. Smyth, and B. Eddie, Chronic relapsing latent meningeal plague, *Arch. Intern. Med.* **59:**967–980 (1937).
87. E. G. H. Koenigsfeld and K. P. S. Nambiar, Plague meningitis, *Indian Med. Gaz.* **81:**474–475 (1946).
88. D. Landsborough and N. Tunnell, Observations on plague meningitis, *Br. Med. J.* **1:**4–7 (1947).
89. E. J. Feeley and J. J. Kriz, Plague meningitis in an American serviceman, *J. Am. Med. Assoc.* **191:**412–413 (1965).
90. A. R. Martin, F. P. Hurtado, R. A. Plessala, E. G. Hurtado, C. E. Chapman, E. L. Callahan, and R. L. Brutsche, Plague meningitis: A report of three cases in children and review of the problem, *Pediatrics* **40:**610–616 (1967).

91. P. D. Tuan, V. Q. Dai, T. T. Ha, and V. Trinh, Meningeal plague: Symposium on Plague, Saigon, October 1970.
92. P. D. Tuan, V. Q. Dai, T. T. Ha, and V. Trinh, Plague meningitis in infants, *Southeast Asian J. Trop. Med. Public Health* **2:**403–405 (1971).
93. M. Isaacson, D. Levy, B. J. Pienaar, H. D. Bubb, J. A. Louv, and D. K. Genis, Unusual cases of human plague in Southern Africa, *S. Afr. Med. J.* **47:**2109–2113 (1973).
94. B. Nilehn, B. Sjostrom, K. Damgaard, and C. Kindmark, *Yersinia enterocolitica* in patients with symptoms of infectious disease, *Acta Pathol. Microbiol. Scand.* **74:**101–113 (1968).
95. C. F. von Reyn, A. M. Barnes, N. S. Weber, T. Quan, and W. J. Dean, Bubonic plague from direct exposure to a naturally infected wild coyote, *Am. J. Trop. Med. Hyg.* **25:**626–629 (1976).

5

Pathogenesis and Toxins

5.1. PLAGUE

5.1.1. Introduction

The pathogenesis of plague has been extensively studied during the past three decades by many dedicated workers at Wilts in England, at Fort Detrick in Maryland, at Walter Reed Army Institute in Washington, D.C., at Albert Einstein University in Philadelphia, and at G.W. Hooper Foundation in San Francisco. By a variety of approaches they sought the mechanisms of disease production by *Yersinia pestis*. They defined certain crucial chemical properties of the plague bacillus that are responsible for its deadly virulence for man and animals. Two general approaches to the problem of virulence were taken by these workers: (1) To identify avirulent mutants of *Y. pestis* and to characterize the defect or missing elements that caused the mutants to have diminished virulence, and (2) to fractionate virulent organisms and to examine culture filtrates for the presence of toxic substances that could mimic the toxicity of whole organisms during natural infections. Recent reviews by Brubaker,[1,2] Walker,[3] and Montie and colleagues[4–6] have discussed some of the important results of these investigations in more detail than I shall in the following sections.

Despite the experimental elegance and biochemical details of these many studies of bacterial virulence, many questions remain unsolved because the properties of the bacteria and of the bacteria–human host relationship that permit the rapid bacterial proliferation have not been fully elucidated. Plague infection is, for the most part, a terrifyingly simple disease to comprehend; there is no need for explanations of subtle biochemical nuance. After the bacteria penetrate the skin, they multiply. Some are phagocytosed by polymorphonuclear leukocytes and macrophages, inside which they multiply further and develop antiphagocyctic properties. Thereafter, the bacilli multiply explosively, with a doubling time of about 2 hr, and gain access to all tissues of the body by circulating in the blood and lymphatic vessels. An acute inflammatory process erupts in the bubo, but the proliferation of organisms continues unabated until a massive density of bacilli, about 10^6–10^{10} bacteria/g of tissue, is attained throughout the body. Inflammatory reactions in many organs, especially in the lymph nodes, liver, and spleen, are intense and destructive, consisting of endothelial damage in blood vessels, hemorrhages, and necrosis. Although rare cases have been described in which tissues of dead patients were sterile, the rule in plague is that death follows an overwhelmingly massive bacterial growth. Therefore, studies seeking to isolate minute quantities of toxic substances that produce metabolic derangements without tissue damage must be viewed critically, lest they lead the researcher to overlook the obvious reality of overwhelming numbers of growing organisms. However, considerable information about the virulence of *Y. pestis* is available.

In susceptible experimental animals, notably mice and guinea pigs, from 1 to 10 viable organisms inoculated subcutaneously will kill the animals after the bacteria have achieved a critical mass of $>10^6$ bacteria/ml of blood. This astonishing mass of bacteria is necessary and sufficient to kill the animals. Avirulent strains of *Y. pestis* fail to achieve uncontrolled bacterial growth to the necessary densities, and certain extracts of great masses of plague bacilli can also kill animals.

5.1.2. Virulence Determinants

Largely from the work of T. W. Burrows and colleagues in England and R. R. Brubaker in the United States, we have gained an understanding of plague virulence. There are at least four phenotypic characters of virulent *Y. pestis* that distinguish this organism from other yersiniae and from most other

TABLE 5.1
Some Phenotypic Differences between Wild-Type *Yersinia pestis* and Other *Yersinia* Species[a]

	Y. pestis	*Y. enterocolitica*	*Y. pseudotuberculosis*
Fraction I (envelope) antigen	+	0	0
Pesticin, coagulase, fibrinolysin	+	0	0
Murine toxin	+	0	0
Pigment formation from chromatophore	+	0	0
Aspartase	0		+
Assimilation of low levels of NH_3	0		+
Cellobiose fermentation	0	+	0
Glucose-6-phosphate dehydrogenase	0		+
Isoleucine/valine biosynthesis	0		+
Methionine biosynthesis	0		+
Melibiose fermentation	0	0	+
Ornithine decarboxylase	0	+	0
Rhamnose fermentation	0	0	+
Sucrose fermentation	0	+	0
Sorbitol fermentation	0	+	0
Threonine/glycine biosynthesis	0		+
Urease	0	+	+
Motility at 26°C	0	+	+

[a] Adapted from R. R. Brubaker[1] in *Microbiology—1979*, with permission of author and publisher.

bacteria as well. These include the production of Fraction I (envelope) antigen, pesticin, murine toxin, and pigment from a chromatophore (Table 5.1). Brubaker has pointed out that other biochemical properties of *Y. pestis* (also listed in Table 5.1) are enzymatic deficiencies that require the plague bacillus to stay within the mammal or flea host almost continuously in order to survive.

By contrast, the other yersiniae possess more enzymatic independence and can survive more competitively in the harsh environment of the bowel or elsewhere in the inanimate environment. Several of the biochemical markers shown in Table 5.1 (including the fermentation of cellobiose, sorbitol, and sucrose) indicate that *Yersinia enterocolitica* may have a more diverse fermentative capability than *Yersinia pseudotuberculosis,* and are useful in the differential laboratory diagnosis of infections due to these yersiniae.

Some of the virulence determinants have been characterized by avirulent mutants that lack the determinants (Table 5.2). They all show a diminished ability to kill mice or guinea pigs that are ordinarily killed by 1 to 10 virulent organisms. Most of the mutants showed only a diminution in virulence, not

TABLE 5.2
Effects of Mutants of *Yersinia pestis* Affecting Virulence Determinants on Lethal Doses for Mice and Guinea Pigs[a]

	Intraperitoneal 50% lethal dose in numbers of bacteria	
	Mice	Guinea pigs
Fully virulent	<10	<10
Mutation causing:		
Lack of V and W antigens	$>10^7$	$>10^8$
Lack of Fraction I (envelope) antigen	<10	10^4
Purine dependence		
Block before inosine monophosphate	10^2	10^4
Block after inosine monophosphate	$>10^7$	$>10^8$
Calcium dependence	$>10^7$	$>10^8$
Lack of pesticin production	10^5	10^6
Lack of pigment production from chromatophore	$>10^7$	$>10^8$

[a] Adapted from R. R. Brubaker in *Microbiology—1979*,[1] with permission of author and publisher.

a total loss of virulence, suggesting that each determinant may act in concert with the others to contribute to full virulence. These data are difficult to apply to man because the virulence of a determinant may vary between species. For example, the absence of Fraction I antigen renders *Y. pestis* less virulent for guinea pigs but not for mice.

5.1.2.1. Fraction I Antigen

This is a glycoprotein, with an estimated molecular weight between 20,000 and 500,000, that is located in the capsular envelope of *Y. pestis* and allows the organism to resist phagocytosis by neutrophils and monocytes. It is produced during growth at 37°C but not at temperatures below 27°C. Thus, organisms proliferating in fleas, which have ambient temperatures, usually do not have a capsule and are relatively susceptible to phagocytosis. After a few cell divisions, however, the progeny of the original inoculum have acquired capsules to resist further phagocytosis. This property of the Fraction

I antigen is widely believed to be the most important single factor and may be a requirement for the uncontrolled surge of bacterial multiplication that characterizes fatal plague infection.

Further work on the chemical composition of the capsular envelope of *Y. pestis* by Glosnicka and Gruszkiewicz[7] showed that a lipid–polysaccharide substance could be extracted from bacteria by suspension in saline. The carbohydrate moieties were galactose and fucose and the lipid constituents phosphatidylethanolamine and phosphatidylserine.

The mechanisms of the antiphagocytic action of Fraction I antigen have been defined by R. C. Williams *et al.* to be interference with the heat-labile opsonins of serum. In particular, the complement components C4 and C2, as well as total hemolytic complement, were consumed when soluble Fraction I was added to serum.[8] Because complement proteins are needed for opsonizing bacteria for efficient phagocytosis, this strong anticomplementary action of Fraction I antigen may explain the resistance of virulent *Y. pestis* to killing by the important host defense mechanisms of phagocytosis.

Caution has been expressed by Brubaker[1] in attributing to Fraction I antigen a preeminent role in virulence. Mutants lacking this antigen still have partial virulence; atypical strains of *Y. pestis* lacking Fraction I antigen have been isolated from patients and animals.[9,10] Nevertheless, this substance has been used to immunize animals against plague, and antiserum directed against Fraction I antigen confers solid immunity against plague.

Another reservation concerning the importance of Fraction I antigen in permitting *Y. pestis* to evade phagocytosis was expressed by Janssen and Surgalla.[11] They showed that both virulent and avirulent organisms grown under conditions that produced bacteria without capsules were capable of surviving inside neutrophils and macrophages after inoculation into the peritoneal cavity of a guinea pig. These intracellular bacteria multiplied within the phagocytes after the cells were removed from animals and observed *in vitro*. Janssen and Surgalla reasoned that the survival and multiplication of bacteria inside phagocytes was more important than resistance to phagocytosis. Actually, the conditions in their experiments may resemble those occurring in nature during the inoculation of *Y. pestis* by fleas when the bacteria lack the antiphagocytic capsules. Only after the initial multiplication inside phagocytes do the organisms develop Fraction I antigen. At a later time in the incubation period, the progeny of the inoculum become resistant to phagocytosis and disseminate from the bubo with abandon throughout the body. This sequence of events is consistent with the results of Cavanaugh and

Randall[12] which show that unencapsulated *Y. pestis* organisms are ingested by leukocytes after inoculation and that neutrophils kill these bacteria but mononuclear phagocytes permit intracellular bacterial multiplication.

5.1.2.2. V and W Antigens

Other antiphagocytic factors that may operate in conjunction with or independent of Fraction I antigen are the V and W antigens, which were discovered by Burrows and Bacon.[13] Avirulent strains lacking Fraction I antigen can develop resistance to phagocytosis by producing V and W antigens. Antisera against these antigens render organisms sensitive to phagocytosis. Lawton *et al.*[14] showed that V is a protein with a molecular weight of 90,000 and W is a lipoprotein with a molecular weight of 145,000.

The V and W antigens of *Y. pestis* are restricted to the cytoplasmic fraction of the bacteria. Straley and Brubaker[15] isolated peptides associated with these virulence determinants by using methods of cell disruption and separation of particles into cytoplasmic and outer-membrane fractions with sucrose gradient centrifugation. By virtue of not being expressed on the cell surface, these antigens probably do not interact directly with host cell membrane surfaces during infection.

The commonly used method for detecting V and W antigens in *Y. pestis* is to streak a culture on agar that contains magnesium oxalate and thus is calcium-free. Virulent bacteria possessing the V and W antigens will not grow at 37°C, whereas avirulent mutants will grow. This nutritional requirement for calcium ions is unique among prokaryotes to the *Yersinia* genus. Zahorchak *et al.*[16] carried out studies of *Y. pestis* grown under calcium-free conditions at 37°C and showed that ribonucleic acid synthesis and protein synthesis were shut off before DNA synthesis. These calcium-deprived cells started growing again when placed into a temperature of 26°C, but the addition of calcium at 37°C after the arrest of growth could not restore growth.

The relevance of the V and W antigens in the pathogenesis of actual infections is uncertain because they are produced by bacteria only during stasis; synthesis of these antigens is suppressed by cell division that occurs in the presence of calcium ions. After phagocytosis, however, these antigens might be synthesized because the cytoplasm of mammalian cells contains insufficient calcium ions to support bacterial division.

5.1.2.3. Purine Dependence

Single-step auxotrophic mutants of *Y. pestis* requiring purines show reduced virulence. Mutant cells blocked by enzyme deficiency at a step in the synthetic pathway prior to inosine monophosphate (IMP) can utilize hypoxanthine for growth and are of only slightly reduced virulence. In contrast, adenine- or guanine-specific mutants blocked after the IMP in the same pathway are innocuous. *In vitro,* the latter could utilize the appropriate purine base, riboside, or deoxyriboside, but not corresponding ribotides or deoxyribotides. These observations indicate that the organisms are unable to transport purine ribotides or deoxyribotides and that insufficient free purines or purine ribosides are available within the host to support growth.

5.1.2.4. Pesticin

Most isolates of *Y. pestis* produce pesticin, a bacteriocin active against serotype I strains of *Y. pseudotuberculosis,* a few isolates of *Y. enterocolitica,* and certain colicin-indicator strains of *Escherichia coli*. Pesticin is a monomeric protein with a molecular weight of about 63,000. It is located in the bacterial cytoplasm. Hall and Brubaker showed that pesticin acts by converting sensitive bacteria to nonviable osmotically stable spheroplasts.[17] The mechanism of action appears to be the enzymatic action of pesticin to hydrolyze mureinlipoproteins in the walls of sensitive bacteria. This enzyme has been defined as *N*-acetylglucosaminidase by Ferber and Brubaker.[18]

The virulence of mutants lacking pesticin is similar to that of wild-type cells introduced to the host by intravenous injection, a route which permits rapid access to fixed macrophages of the liver and spleen.[19] In contrast, these mutants show reduced virulence when injected by peripheral routes, thus revealing an inability to invade deep tissues of the host. Pesticin itself probably does not facilitate dissemination. This process apparently is caused by distinct envelope-associated fibrinolytic and coagulase activities that accompany pesticin production. Spontaneous mutation to a pesticin-negative state results in loss of the fibrinolysin and coagulase, suggesting that these components are expressed as a function of bacteriocinogenic conversion.[20] Peptides corresponding to the fibrinolysin and coagulase have been localized by Straley and Brubaker[15] to the outer membrane fraction of bacterial cells.

Virulence of pesticin-negative mutant cells is increased in mice receiving sufficient Fe^{3+} by injection to saturate serum transferrin. The injected iron probably inhibits H_2O_2-dependent killing mechanisms of professional phagocytes rather than having a direct enhancing action on the bacteria themselves. This inhibition of phagocytic killing in the tissues may allow mutant organisms to reach favored sites and to proliferate in the liver and spleen.[(19)]

Wake and co-workers[(20)] showed the virulence of an avirulent strain of *Y. pestis* (EV, line NIIEG) also could be increased in mice by treating the mice with the colloidal iron chondroitin sulfate. Their results indicated that the colloidal iron interfered with host defense mechanisms. It is likely that the iron particles produced a blockade of the reticuloendothelial system, thus preventing fixed macrophages of the spleen, liver, and bone marrow from effectively phagocytosing disseminated bacteria during acute infection.

5.1.2.5. Pigment Production

Virulent *Y. pestis* strains absorb certain exogenous planar low-molecular-weight chromatophores and will grow as pigmented colonies on semisolid media. Mutants unable to produce pigment have reduced virulence, which (like the pesticin-negative mutants) can be overcome by injecting mice with iron. Brubaker[(19)] has suggested that the injected iron in this case may act directly on the bacteria to restore virulence, because hemin has been shown to promote the production of pigment. This restoration could occur in strains that were previously pigment-negative.

The significance of pigment production appears to be that it is a mechanism for the bacteria to extract iron, an essential element for growth, from the environment. Since *Y. pestis* cannot synthesize its own iron-absorbing chromatophores, it must acquire these chromatophores from other bacteria or from host sources. Then, *Y. pestis* has an important biological advantage of being able to proliferate in animal tissues where iron exists in low, growth-limiting concentrations. The availability of iron and perhaps other metallic ions has been suggested by Rail[(21)] to be a critical environmental factor for the occurrence of plague infection in any given region.

5.1.3. Determinants of Pathogenicity

The virulence determinants discussed in the previous section are properties of the *Y. pestis* that allow the organism to establish itself in the host tissues after inoculation by permitting it to survive, to multiply, and to become disseminated. These virulence determinants appear to act by neutralizing certain antibacterial defense mechanisms of the host, such as phagocytosis and intracellular bacterial killing by enzymatic degradation.

The determinants of pathogenicity differ from the virulence determinants in that they are toxins which produce tissue injury in the host after bacteria have proliferated to achieve the high critical density in host tissues. Although the biochemical characteristics of the determinants of virulence and pathogenicity may be interrelated and, in some cases, may be even the same chemical substances, the traditional view which I have taken in this chapter is that the mechanisms of virulence operate during the incubation period and thus precede those of pathogenicity, which are expressed during the actual disease.

There are two major categories of toxins in plague that have been incriminated as determinants of pathogenicity. The endotoxin of plague is a structural component of the cell wall and resembles closely the lipopolysaccharide endotoxin of other gram-negative bacteria. The exotoxin(s) of plague, on the other hand, are enzymatic proteins secreted by the bacteria and are unique to *Y. pestis*.

5.1.3.1. Endotoxin

a. Structure of the Lipopolysaccharide Molecule. In 1956, Davies[22] described the chemical composition of lipopolysaccharide (LPS) extracted by hot phenol and water from *Y. pestis*. This material was free of protein and nucleic acids and contained glucose, glucoseamine, and an aldoheptose sugar, which composed the greater part of the carbohydrate moiety. This sugar was subsequently shown by Foster *et al.*[23] to be L-glycero-D-mannoheptose. The chemical similarity of the LPS of *Y. pestis* to the LPS of *E. coli* was shown in 1968 by Ellwood[24] who identified 3-deoxy-D-manno-octulosonic acid (KDO) as a glycosidic component of the LPS of the bacteria. KDO now is known to be present in the LPS molecules extracted from all Enterobacteriaceae and is a vital part of the so-called core region of the LPS. A closely related or identical sugar component has been found in other bacterial LPS and is called 2-keto-3-deoxyoctonate, also referred to as KDO.

The lipid portion of the LPS of *Y. pestis* was studied in 1966 by Walker *et al.*[25] After alkaline hydrolysis of LPS, thin layer chromatography revealed a cephalinlike band that resembled phosphatidyl ethanolamine. Further studies of lipids by Hartley *et al.*[26] identified Lipid A in the LPS of *Y. pestis*. The importance of Lipid A is that this material is the toxic portion of the LPS derived from all other gram-negative bacteria. The Lipid A of *Y. pestis* was composed of glucoseamine, glucoseamine-6-phosphate, and ethanolamine, with only one principal fatty acid, β-hydroxymyristate. The molecular model of Lipid A of other LPS preparations consists of a backbone of phosphorylated glucoseamine units with β-hydroxymyristate linked to the amino groups of glucoseamine and other fatty acids linked to the hydroxyl groups of glucoseamine. Hartley *et al.*[26] suggests that this model is applicable to the LPS of *Y. pestis,* but the structure of this LPS appeared simpler than other LPS by virtue of β-hydroxymyristate being predominant and other ester-linked fatty acids being present in small amounts.

Native LPS of *Y. pestis* is highly aggregated, and thus, the molecular weight has been difficult to estimate. Hartley *et al.*[26] calculated the particle weight of phenol-extracted LPS to be 1.6×10^8 daltons by sedimentation velocity. In the ultracentrifuge, the LPS sedimented at 29,500 rpm, and when examined by electron microscopy, this preparation of LPS consisted of thread-like structures that were about 8 nm in diameter.

b. Function of Plague Endotoxin. Prior to 1956, when Davies[22] first extracted a biologically active LPS from *Y. pestis* using a hot phenol–water method, it was believed that the plague bacillus did not contain LPS, perhaps because the organism is surrounded by the thick Fraction I protein capsule. Davies showed that his LPS was pyrogenic in rabbits and lethal to mice, but was considerably less potent on a weight basis than LPS of other Enterobacteriaceae. Subsequent studies with LPS of *Y. pestis* have established that this material possesses the whole range of pathogenic and biological effects that characterize other gram-negative bacterial LPS, including a biphasic fever pattern in rabbits, lethal shock in animals with vascular damage and hemorrhage in kidneys, liver, and other organs,[27,28] localized and generalized Shwartzman reactions in rabbits,[29] gelation of limulus lysate, and mitogenic stimulation of B lymphocytes of the murine spleen.[30] Like pathogenic and biological effects due to LPS extracted from other gram-negative bacteria, these activities could be inhibited by exposing the LPS to the antibiotic polymyxin.[30] In humans with plague infection, endotoxin has been detected by bioassays in mice[31] and by the limulus test,[32] and lesions of characteristic endotoxin pathophysiology have been noted. Finegold showed that glomerular blood vessels in the kidneys of fatal cases of plague contained fibrin thrombi, which resembled the generalized Shwartzman reaction in rabbits that were injected with endotoxin.[33]

The mechanisms by which plague endotoxin produces disease and tissue damage are not fully understood. The subject of endotoxin pathophysiology has been a large and diverse area of active investigation during recent years. Many cells and tissues of the body will respond to endotoxin, and these include phagocytic cells of the blood, liver, and spleen, lymphocytes, and blood platelets. Plasma proteins, including the complement proteins and Hageman factor, are activated also by endotoxin, resulting in intravascular coagulation, the production of mediators of hypotension, and chemotaxis of leukocytes into areas of inflammation. Two of the prominent disease characteristics in plague infection, fever and intravascular coagulation, may be the result of the activation of mononuclear phagocytic cells by endotoxin. These cells include both blood monocytes and the fixed macrophages in the reticuloendothelial system of the lymph nodes, liver, spleen, and bone marrow. All of these tissues contain plentiful bacteria during plague infection and so it is a reasonable possibility that plague endotoxin may be operative at these sites. The mononuclear phagocytes, when exposed to endotoxin, begin to synthesize and secrete large quantities of both leukocytic pyrogen,[34] which acts on the hypothalamus to elevate body temperature, and tissue thromboplastin,[35,36] an enzyme which triggers the activation of the cascade of clotting proteins resulting in the formation of fibrin clots.

The local and generalized Shwartzman reactions in rabbits are relevant to the pathology caused by plague endotoxin. For the local Shwartzman reaction, endotoxin is first injected intradermally and 24 hr later an intravenous injection of endotoxin is given. Within 6 hr after the intravenous injection, the skin site of the first injection shows hemorrhagic necrosis with pathology revealing both thrombosis of blood vessels with fibrin and the resulting hemorrhagic infarction of the skin. In the generalized Shwartzman reaction, two intravenous injections of sublethal doses of endotoxin are administered 24 hr apart. The first injection is called the preparation dose, the second the provoking dose. Six hours or longer after the provoking dose, the kidneys show cortical necrosis and hemorrhagic infarction due to intravascular coagulation in the glomerular arterioles and larger arteries. Similar vascular lesions are present in other tissues. Recent work by Bohn and Muller-Berghaus[37] using leukopenic rabbits suggests that the preparation for the generalized Shwartzman reaction is caused by endothelial cell damage in blood vessels and that the provoking of the reaction is caused by a leukocyte-mediated acceleration of intravascular blood clotting.

In 1937, Koplik performed some beautiful experiments demonstrating that lymph nodes can be the target of a local Shwartzman reaction following injection of endotoxin into the skin.[38] Culture filtrates of *Salmonella typhi* were injected by the intradermal or intralymphatic route and 24 hr later intravenously. The lymph nodes draining the skin sites, as well as the skin sites, showed hemorrhage and necrosis. The regional lymph nodes, but not the more distant nodes, were enlarged with gross hemorrhage. The microscopic examination revealed endothelial cell swelling, thrombosis of blood vessels, and plentiful polymorphonuclear leukocytes and macrophages. A single intradermal or intralymphatic injection of culture filtrates did not produce this lesion, nor did a single intravenous injection.

The similarity of the histology of lymph nodes in the local Shwartzman reaction as demonstrated by Koplik and the histology of buboes in plague infection indicates that a similar pathophysiology is operative. In plague infection, the host is inoculated intradermally with bacteria containing endotoxin. There may be some bacterial multiplication at the skin site, and bacteria are transported by lymphatic vessels to the regional lymph nodes where further multiplication occurs. Thus, the lymph node becomes "prepared" for a local Shwartzman reaction. At the onset of clinical illness, patients have fever and chills, often with bacteremia and endotoxemia. At this time, the provoking of the reaction occurs. The bubo swells and develops its characteristic hemorrhagic necrosis. Occasionally, patients will manifest skin eschars or ulcerations, indicating that local cutaneous Shwartzman reactions may also occur. The widespread cutaneous necrosis and gangrene that have been described in plague and are the basis of the epithet "black death" are likely to be also the result of a generalized Shwartzman reaction in which cutaneous blood vessels were principally the target tissues of the endotoxin exposure.

Other biological effects of plague endotoxin that may be relevant to human infections have been demonstrated by Walker[25,28] in experimental animals (Table 5.3). These are the metabolic effects of depletion of liver glycogen, decrease in blood sugar, and elevation of blood urea nitrogen. Endotoxin may produce these effects by impairing kidney function and by altering carbohydrate metabolism through a stress reaction mediated by epinephrine. The pathology of animals revealed renal tubular damage and fatty infiltration of liver cells. In fatal human cases of plague examined by Finegold,[33] the kidneys frequently showed intravascular coagulation and cortical necrosis that resembled the lesions of the generalized Shwartzman reaction in rabbits.

The relevance of plague endotoxin to human disease was further established by Butler *et al.*[32] using the limulus test, a new assay for endotoxin.

TABLE 5.3
Some Determinants of Virulence and Pathogenicity in *Yersinia pestis*

Name	Chemical nature	Mol. wt.	Biological importance	Location in bacterium	LD50 in mice	Mechanism of action
Fraction I antigen	Glycoprotein	20,000–500,000	Antiphagocytic against polymorphonuclear leukocytes	Capsular envelope	—	Depletes serum of complement proteins, especially C2, C4
V and W antigens						
V	Protein	90,000	Antiphagocytic and produced by static bacteria	Cell wall	—	Unknown
W	Lipoprotein	145,000				
Pesticin	Protein	65,000	May allow to compete for survival in nature by inhibiting growth of other bacteria	Unknown	—	Kills other yersiniae and some *E. coli* by converting them to osmotically stable spheroplasts
Endotoxin	Lipopolysaccharide	1.6×10^8 of particle aggregates	Mediator of fever, shock, intravascular coagulation	Cytoplasm	300–500 μg	In mice depletes liver glycogen, lowers blood sugar, raises blood urea nitrogen
Murine toxin					0.1–3 μg	
Toxin A	Protein	240,000	Unknown	Cytoplasmic membrane, cytoplasm	1 μg	β-adrenergic antagonism, in high concentrations causes mitochondrial swelling, inhibits oxidation of α-keto acids, and prevents reduction of coenzyme Q
Toxin B	Protein	120,000	Unknown		8 μg	

This test is the most sensitive method for detecting endotoxin in body fluids, capable of detecting as little as 0.0001 μg/ml, which corresponds to about 10^3 bacteria/ml when whole bacteria are the only source of endotoxin. The test is based on the ability of endotoxin to produce coagulation of soluble clottable proteins in the granules of amebocytes from the hemolymph of the horseshoe crab (*Limulus polyphemus*). Patients with acute bubonic plague in Vietnam frequently had endotoxemia detected by the limulus test, but the same patients after recovery had negative blood tests for endotoxin. Endotoxin was also detectable in the spinal fluid of patients with plague meningitis. Thus, the detection of endotoxin in body fluids of patients with plague and the presence of symptoms and specific pathology in patients that can be experimentally elicited by endotoxin strongly implicates this biologically active substance in having a large role in the pathogenesis of plague.

5.1.3.2. Plague Exotoxin

Another substance that is produced by *Y. pestis* has competed with endotoxin for the attention of investigators. This substance is the soluble protein toxin which is called the murine toxin because it is highly lethal for mice but less lethal for other animal species. Review papers by Walker in 1967,[3] Kadis *et al.* in 1966,[39] Montie *et al.* in 1975[5] and Montie in 1981[6] have amply detailed information on this substance. In this section, I will summarize certain aspects of the plague toxin, discuss the more recently recognized β-adrenergic blocking activity of toxin, and make conclusions about the relevance of the toxin in human disease.

a. Structure. The murine toxin is a protein contained within the bacterial cytoplasmic membrane. By the technique of continuous-flow paper electrophoresis, the toxin has been separated into two proteins that are called Toxin A and Toxin B. Toxin A has a molecular weight of 240,000 and Toxin B has one of 120,000 (Table 5.3). Toxin B contains significantly less tryptophan than Toxin A. Both toxins could be dissociated by treatment with sodium dodecyl sulfate into subunits with molecular weights between 12,000 and 24,000, and these subunits retained most of the toxicity of the parent toxin.

Both toxin proteins have a high content of acidic amino acids and a low content of cysteine residues. Chemical alterations of toxin molecules indicated that both sulfhydryl groups and tryptophan residues were essential for toxicity.[5,40,41] The specific toxin activity by weight was higher for Toxin A than Toxin B.

b. Biological Activity of Murine Toxin. First, the toxin was shown to inhibit respiration of mitochondria in cells from the heart of the toxin-susceptible mouse and rat, but not that of mitochondria in cells from similar tissues of the toxin-resistant rabbit, dog, monkey, and chimpanzee.[42] In the living toxin-susceptible animal, injection of the toxin produced electrocardiographic changes in the S-T segment, suggesting that the effect on heart mitochondria could be clinically relevant. Within the mitochondrion, the biochemical action of the toxin was shown to be inhibition of the electron transfer system at the step of Complex I, which is prior to coenzyme Q. The enzyme in this sequence that was inhibited by the toxin was shown to be reduced nicotinamide adenine dinucleotide-coenzyme Q reductase. Additionally, the toxin inhibited the uptake of calcium and inorganic phosphate ions by susceptible heart mitochondria by inducing the mitochondria to swell. In these experiments, a disturbing finding was the requirement of very high concentrations of toxin, 0.5–2.0 mg/ml, to block mitochondrial respiration. This must be compared to the small quantities of toxin, 0.1–3 μg, required to kill a 20-g mouse, and raises the possibility that the high-dose effect was not biologically relevant.

Studies by Hildebrand *et al.*[43] showed that animals intoxicated with plague murine toxin did not die from heart failure but from peripheral circulatory collapse. Thus, Montie and co-workers[5,44] sought other possible mechanisms of action of the plague toxin, which led to the concept that plague toxin is a hormonal antagonist of β-adrenergic activity and probably also an antagonist of cyclic adenosine 3^1, 5^1-monophosphate (cAMP). Beginning with the observation that mice that are injected with 3 μg of toxin showed decreased blood levels of glucose and free fatty acids, they postulated that the toxin exerted an insulinlike effect. Measurement of insulin activity in blood during intoxication, however, showed normal levels. Treatment of intoxicated mice with glucose or epinephrine did not reverse toxicity, but the simultaneous administration of dibutryl cAMP, glucagon, or cortisone with toxin resulted in reduced toxicity. Furthermore, the effect of epinephrine to elevate blood glucose and free fatty acid concentration in blood was blocked by the toxin. Thus, the murine toxin appeared to produce a β-adrenergic blockade.

The mechanism of this β-adrenergic blockade was further studied by Brown and Montie.[44] When cholera toxin is injected into animals, it produces an elevation of cAMP in nearly all cells of the body by activation of the enzyme adenylate cyclase. The administration of cholera toxin to mice at the same time that a lethal dose of plague toxin was given caused a reversal of lethal toxicity. Dibutryl cAMP also antagonized the lethal effect of plague toxin. Whereas the plague toxin prevented the rise in plasma free fatty acids produced by epinephrine, the rise in plasma free fatty acids produced by dibutryl cAMP was not prevented by toxin. Epinephrine and other β-adrenergic agonists act on many cells of the body that possess β-adrenergic receptors to produce elevations in intracellular cAMP. Because plague toxin blocks the action of epinephrine but not that of cAMP, it appears that the plague toxin antagonizes β-adrenergic activity at a site in the pathway before adenylate cyclase. Further evidence for the activity of the murine toxin on cAMP was obtained by Montie[6] in experiments with mice that received anti-cAMP antiserum, and the mice demonstrated enhanced susceptibility to the toxin.

5.1.3.3. Opposing Views of Toxins of *Yersinia pestis*

It has not been entirely resolved whether the endotoxin or murine toxin of *Y. pestis* plays a dominant role in actual plague infections. It has been pointed out that both toxins may act together synergistically and that some activities, such as hypoglycemia in mice, are produced by either toxin.

The weight of evidence appears to favor the dominant role of endotoxin. Human disease is characterized by typical symptoms and signs attributable to endotoxin. These include fever, hypotension, disseminated intravascular coagulation, the local Shwartzman reaction (bubo), and the generalized Shwartzman reaction. Walker has further shown that the lethal doses of endotoxin are more consistently toxic for several species of animals than are doses of murine toxin.[3] This universal toxicity of endotoxin suggests that man is more likely to be affected by endotoxin than by the murine toxin.

Additional arguments for the dominant role of endotoxin concern quantitative relationships between bacterial mass and endotoxin. From lethal dose experiments in guinea pigs, Walker has estimated that the 50% lethal dose (LD50) is about 1300 mg of acetone-killed whole bacteria/kg of animal weight.[3] The LD50 of endotoxin was 83–165 mg/kg for guinea pigs, or about 10% that of whole bacteria. The amount of purified endotoxin that Davies extracted from *Y. pestis* was 2% of the starting bacterial weight. These figures of 10%

and 2%, which are in the comparable range, indicate the plausibility that a sizeable portion of the bacterial weight that consists of endotoxin provides the necessary toxin to kill animals. Furthermore, during a natural infection of mice, death occurs when bacteria have densely populated the tissues in numbers as high as 10^9/g. Thus, a dead mouse may contain about 10^{10} bacteria, which may weigh about 10 mg and from which about 2% of the weight, or 200 μg, could be extracted as endotoxin. This is approximately a lethal dose of endotoxin for a mouse.[(45)] Therefore, dying animals with plague infection have enough endotoxin present in their bodies to explain their lethality. Such quantitative relationships between whole bacteria and extracted murine toxin have not been developed.

Walker has also related the heat stability of endotoxin to lethality. Heating whole bacteria to 100°C did not decrease the LD50 of whole bacteria for guinea pigs. Endotoxin is heat stable, whereas the murine toxin is heat labile. Thus, the lethality of whole organisms is better explained by endotoxin.[(3)] Other problems with the concept of the murine toxin indicate that it may not be relevant biologically. The murine toxin is part of the bacterial membrane and may not be released from bacteria to reach distant target cells of the host. It has not been measured in blood or other tissues of infected patients or animals in the same manner that endotoxin has been assayed. The described activity on heart mitochondria required very high concentrations of toxin. Furthermore, the β-adrenergic blocking action of the toxin has been described only in mice, which have a carbohydrate metabolism that differs greatly from that of other species. For example, cortisone can reverse endotoxin lethality in mice by preventing hypoglycemia, but this effect cannot be so easily observed in other species.

Another conceptual problem with all toxins in plague infection is whether any putative toxins in this disease act like hormones at sites distant from the actual foci of multiplying bacteria. Plague is characterized by enormous numbers of bacteria which elicit raging destructive inflammatory reactions. From this great quantity of bacteria and inflammatory cell products, it may be conceptually incorrect to seek minute quantities of a potent bacterial biochemical poison that can act "cleanly" on host cell metabolism to produce enzymatic blockades. Table 5.4 contrasts the effects of endotoxin and murine toxin in the mouse with the effects of actual infection with living bacteria. Intoxication with each toxin produces some but not all the effects of experimental infections, indicating that neither toxin can duplicate the actions of bacterial infection.

TABLE 5.4
Effects of Plague Toxins Compared to Effects of Infection on Physiology of the Mouse

	Murine toxin	Endotoxin	Infection with *Y. pestis*
50% lethal dose	0.1–3 μg	300–10,000 μg	⩾1 organism injected proliferates to more than 10^9–10^{10} per mouse
Time of death after injection	8–9 hr	12–15 hr	2–8 days depending on inoculum
Pathology	Minor vascular damage in brain, lungs, peritoneum	Severe vascular damage and hemorrhage in many organs	Many bacteria in vessels with hemorrhage and thrombosis and necrosis of many organs
Blood sugar	Hypoglycemia	Hypoglycemia	Unknown
Blood urea nitrogen	Unknown	Azotemia	Unknown

5.1.3.4. Plasmids of *Yersinia pestis*

One of the most significant advances of bacterial genetics in the decade of 1970s was the recognition that plasmids frequently are present in pathogenic bacteria. These small extrachromosomal pieces of DNA replicate independently of the chromosomal DNA and can be transferred from one bacterial cell to another during a mating procedure. Plasmids which encode antibiotic resistance are called R factors but other plasmids are known to encode many virulence factors of pathogenic bacteria.

Plasmids in several strains of *Y. pestis* obtained from different countries have been identified by Ferber and Brubaker using electrophoresis in agarose gels.[(46)] The absence of certain of these plasmids is associated with loss of virulence determinants and accordingly these plasmids have been assigned the important role of providing directly to the bacterium the genetic information that is necessary to direct the synthesis of certain proteins that confer virulence to *Y. pestis* (Table 5.5).

This recent discovery of plasmids in *Y. pestis* has profound significance for understanding the biology of this organism because it allows a reinter-

TABLE 5.5
Plasmids of *Yersinia pestis* Controlling Virulence

Virulence determinant	Plasmid character
V and W antigens and calcium dependency	45 megadalton
Pesticin	6 megadalton
Murine toxin	65 megadalton (cryptic)
Java strain (no known virulence determinant)[a]	20 megadalton

[a] This plasmid was found in the Java strain but confers no known virulence determinant to the organism.

pretation of certain evolutionary and laboratory events. The acquisition of virulence determinants by *Y. pestis* was supposed to be the result of random genetic mutation, followed by Darwinian natural selection of those mutants that improved survivability and multiplication of the bacterium in the environment and its natural hosts. Now we must consider that these virulence determinants could have been more rapidly acquired by plasmid transfer from other bacteria. Conversely, these plasmid-mediated virulence determinants could be transferred from *Y. pestis* to other bacteria, such as to other yersiniae or other Enterobacteriaciae, and these other bacteria could assume some of the virulence properties of the plague bacillus.

The laboratory phenomenon of attenuation of virulence by serial passage of bacteria in culture media can also be reinterpreted in the light of the newly recognized plasmids. Many plasmids are known to be lost spontaneously from bacteria during laboratory passage. Thus, vaccine strains of *Y. pestis* produced in this manner and lacking in virulence are likely to be plasmidless strains rather than true mutants. Similarly, some atypical strains of *Y. pestis* isolated from people or animals that lack certain features of the typical strains are probably the result of plasmid loss.

The evolutionary significance of virulence plasmids in *Y. pestis* is that plasmids conferred genetic advantage to the plague bacillus. The obvious advantage was that bacteria which possessed the plasmid-mediated attributes could successfully counter host defense mechanisms and permit unbridled multiplication of bacteria. An evolutionary disadvantage of the virulence factors was that "unnatural hosts" like man were killed quickly by bacteria and further propagation of bacteria could not occur. But in better-adapted animal hosts, these virulence factors and perhaps other factors allowed bacteria to multiply without killing the host.

A minor evolutionary disadvantage of plasmid acquisition, which is overcome by the larger advantage of bacterial survivability in host tissues, is the genetic burden of additional information that must be translated into protein synthesis through the use of energy-requiring enzymatic steps. This is perhaps the reason that plasmids are lost during laboratory passage where bacteria do not need to oppose the forces of host tissue defenses. Likewise, R factor plasmids are often lost when bacteria are removed from environments with antibiotic pressure.

5.1.3.5. Experimental Infections

In the original descriptions of the plague bacillus given independently in 1894 by Yersin and Kitasato (See Chapter 2), these scientists injected a variety of animals with bacterial cultures and demonstrated the remarkable lethality of *Y. pestis*. In general, mice and guinea pigs are highly susceptible to fatal infections, whereas rats, rabbits, and squirrels are more resistant. Carnivores are also relatively resistant, but will die if they ingest large inocula of organisms. In this section, I have selected only two experimental approaches to plague infection which explore infection by aerosol inhalation and by ingestion.

a. Plague Infection of Lungs by Aerosols. Plague pneumonias can be transmitted by infected airborne droplets and are very lethal to man. Finegold and co-workers infected rhesus monkeys with aerosols of *Y. pestis* in order to study the mechanisms of pathogenicity.[47,48] They exposed monkeys to aerosols made by a nebulizer that produced aerosol particles with a mean diameter of 1.25 μm. Each monkey inhaled a mean inoculum of 3×10^4 viable *Y. pestis* organisms. After an incubation period that ranged from 2–5 days, monkeys became suddenly ill with tachypnea and prostration. Fever appeared on the 4th or 5th day. Death occurred commonly between 3 and 7 days after exposure.

Blood coagulation studies were carried out daily to look for changes of disseminated intravascular coagulation. At the early period of 1–2 days after exposure, monkeys showed abnormalities that consisted of prolonged clotting times, partial thromboplastin times, and prothrombin times and decreased platelet counts. The fibrinogen levels, however, showed increases. These results indicated that disseminated intravascular coagulation was a common early event in plague pneumonia.

All stages of pneumonia were seen within the lungs of animals that died. Foci of lobular consolidation were found in the peripheral portion of single lobes, most often a lower lobe. They consisted of an area 0.5–3 cm in diameter of firm purple tissue between the central bronchovascular trunk and the pleura. On section, there was hepatization, occasionally with central liquefaction and hemorrhage. The surrounding tissue was edematous, often for a greater area than the consolidation portion. Edema fluid was sometimes present in a second lobe. At most, less than half of pulmonary tissue was involved. Microscopically, advanced lesions consisted of a central abscess. Hemorrhages were common and inflamed vessels frequent in such areas. Lesser reactions consisted of alveolar consolidation of polymorphonuclear leukocytes with intact septums. At the margins of the pneumonia, alveoli were filled with edema fluid teeming with bacilli which had the bipolar staining typical of *Y. pestis*. Similar areas of alveolar edema without leukocytic infiltration were common in secondary lesions in less involved lobes, presumably arising from intrabronchial dissemination. Dilatation of lymphatics around bronchi and veins was common in areas of edematous alveoli. The lymphatics were also heavily colonized by bacteria. Fibrin was notably absent from the exudate at all stages, but intravascular thrombi were sometimes seen.

Bronchial lymph nodes that drained the infected lobes displayed extensive liquefaction necrosis in all animals. Large numbers of bacilli were present. Hemorrhages were also numerous.

In the spleen a reduction in cellularity of the red pulp was common, with hemorrhages and foci of necrosis in some cases. Usually bacilli were abundant, and, sometimes, fibrin was found in the sinusoids. There were a few instances of increased numbers of polymorphonuclear leukocytes. The lymphoid tissue was generally unaffected.

In the liver, lesions were generally minimal and included sinusoidal congestion, periportal or diffuse sinusoidal leukocytosis, and mild fatty change. Bacilli and fibrin were ocasionally found in sinusoids.

The kidneys in 20 of 25 autopsied monkeys showed fibrin thrombi in the glomerular capillaries. In cases with extensive deposits, some afferent arterioles and intertubular and medullary capillaries were also occluded. Cortical necrosis was seen in some of the kidneys with extensive thrombosis. With fewer thrombi, the parenchymal changes were limited to focal glomerular hypercellularity and vacuolar degeneration of proximal tubular epithelium. Pale eosinophilic fluid occasionally was present in Bowman's space and the proximal tubular lumen. The fibrin was readily seen in hematoxylin–eosin-stained sections as homogeneous hyaline material. In Giemsa-stained sections, bacilli were found in a small proportion of the thrombi. The phosphotungstic-acid–hematoxylin stain and electron microscopy confirmed that the thrombi were composed of fibrin.

The possibility that these observations are limited to a specific strain of *Y. pestis* or to the aerosol route of inoculation was considered. Sections from a previous experiment were examined. Seven rhesus monkeys had been given subcutaneous injections of 3×10^9 bacilli of the Alexander strain. They lived an average of 85.6 hr, and displayed typical bubonic plague: local ulceration and liquefactive necrosis of the subcutaneous tissue at the site of inoculation, inguinal buboes composed of necrotic lymph nodes, septicemia with abundant intravascular bacilli in all organs, and multiple hemorrhages. Fibrin thrombi were extensive in the glomerular capillaries of six of seven animals.

These observations of monkeys with experimental plague pneumonia suggest that plague pneumonia is a rapidly fatal disease, not only because of the fulminant local disease in the lungs, but also because of the systemic effects. Widespread infection was present in dying monkeys in the blood stream, kidneys, spleen, and liver. Furthermore, this experimental model provides further evidence for the role of plague endotoxin in the pathogenesis of this infection. Animals displayed marked signs of disseminated intravascular coagulation and fibrin deposition in renal glomeruli, both of which are part of the generalized Shwartzman reaction in rabbits, which is experimentally produced by injections of endotoxin.

b. Plague Infections of Rodents by the Oral Route. In this section, I will describe an approach to understanding how plague infection may be transmitted by ingestion in addition to the more commonly accepted route of infected flea bites (Butler *et al.*[48a]). In 1894, Yersin first showed that rats and mice could be fatally infected by feeding them fragments of spleen or liver from animals that had died with plague. Although rodents are not naturally carnivores, they eat dead litter-mates in capitivity and may do so occasionally in their natural burrows. Natural carnivores such as bobcats, coyotes, and cats can develop fatal systematic infections with plague after ingesting infected rodents, and these carnivores have transmitted plague to humans (e.g., hunters) who have handled the animals. The implication that *Y. pestis* could have a larger role in the intestinal niche than has been previously appreciated may be derived from its classification in the family Enterobacteriaceae.

In order to compare the infectivity of *Y. pestis* by the intragastric and subcutaneous routes, different groups of rodents received graded doses of *Y. pestis* by both routes. Intragastric inoculations were given by a No. 16 feeding cannula attached to a syringe. All dead rodents were autopsied and had positive organ cultures. Surviving rodents were sacrificed and those with positive organ cultures or with titers of passive hemagglutination antibody against Fraction IA $\geqslant 16$ were added to those that died with positive organ cultures to obtain infective doses. As shown in Table 5.6, all three species were susceptible to fatal infection with *Y. pestis* by the intragastric route. Of the two Brazilian rodent species inoculated with the same strain of *Y. pestis*, *Rattus rattus* was more resistant to infection than was *Zygodontomys pixuna*. The 50% infective dose (ID50) values for *Mus musculus* (CF-1 mice) and *Rattus rattus* were lower than the LD50 values because some of these rodents showed serological responses to infection. For all species the subcutaneous route produced LD50 and ID50 values that were at least 1000-fold lower than the corresponding values obtained for intragastric inoculation. The values of 0.7 ($\log_{10} = -0.15$) bacteria for the LD50 and ID50 for mice by the subcutaneous routes demonstrated both the high susceptibility of these rodents and the virulence of *Y. pestis* for this species that permitted one bacterium to kill some of the mice (Table 5.6). Most deaths occurred between 3 and 8 days after inoculation.

TABLE 5.6
Susceptibility of Rodents to *Yersinia pestis* Infection by the Intragastric and Subcutaneous Routes[a]

	Intragastric		Subcutaneous	
	LD50	ID50	LD50	ID50
M. musculus[b]	6.32	5.04	−0.15	−0.15
Z. pixuna[c]	5.46	5.46	1.73	1.46
R. rattus	9.62	7.26	6.62	3.30

[a] Numbers are the $\log_{10}$ viable bacteria that were the 50% lethal doses (LD50) and 50% infective doses (ID50) calculated by the method of Reed and Muench.

[b] CF-1 laboratory mice were inoculated with a strain of *Y. pestis* isolated in Vietnam.

[c] *Z. pixuna* and *R. rattus* trapped in rural Brazil were inoculated with a strain of *Y. pestis* isolated in Brazil.

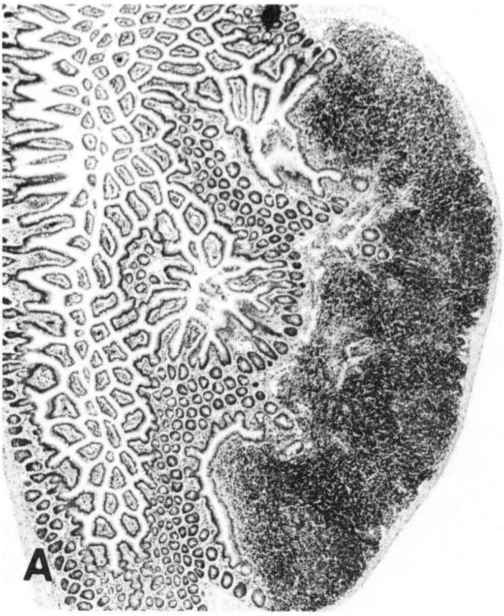

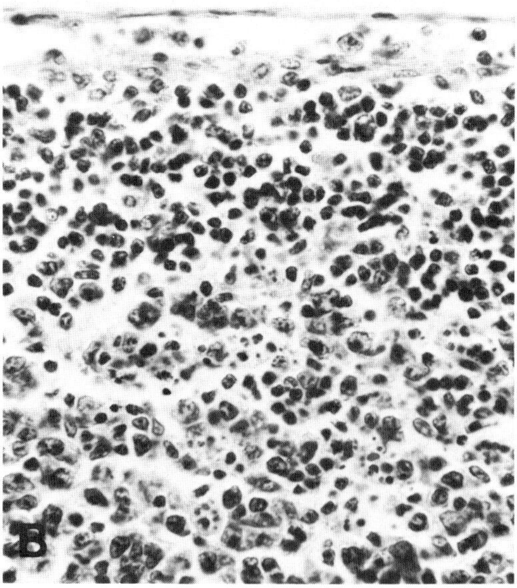

FIGURE 5.1. Characteristic pathological changes in CF-1 mice with fatal *Y. pestis* infection acquired by intragastric inoculation. (A) In the terminal ileum a Peyer's patch shows lymphoid hyperplasia. The mucosa overlying the Peyer's patch and villi is intact. Magnification × 31. (B) A mesenteric lymph node shows increased numbers of mononuclear cells. Magnification × 320. (C) A section of liver shows microabcesses with collection of neutrophils (arrow). Magnification × 400. (D) The red pulp of a spleen shows extensive necrosis and neutrophilic infiltration. Macrophages (arrow) and massive numbers of extracellular bacteria are present (arrowhead). Magnification × 320.

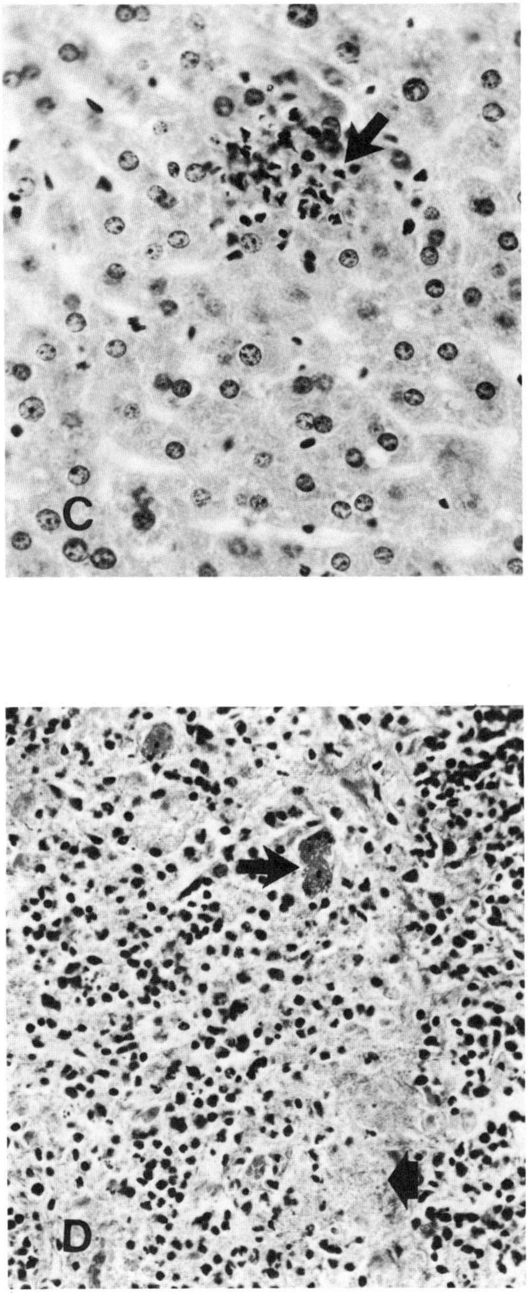
C
D

Early deaths occurred usually in those animals that received the largest inocula.

To determine whether *Y. pestis* was also virulent when naturally ingested, bacterial suspensions were prepared from colonies on a chocolate agar plate and diluted with distilled water to a final concentration of about 10^8 organisms/ml. Five mice were allowed to drink 20 ml of infected water. All died 3 days later and smears and cultures of tissues revealed heavy *Y. pestis* infection.

Gross and microscopic pathologic examinations were made of 10 mice infected either by intragastric inoculation or by permitted ingestion of water that contained bacteria. Animals were selected that were moribund or freshly dead, and infection with *Y. pestis* was confirmed by positive spleen, liver, and blood cultures. Gross and microscopic examinations of lungs revealed no evidence of pneumonia. Thus, aspiration of bacteria either from the stomachs or during drinking was excluded as a mechanism for the introduction of bacteria across mucosal surfaces. The spleens were moderately enlarged. The small intestines did not show changes of enteritis or abcess formation. Microscopically, most animals had minimal changes of increased mitosis of intestinal epithelial cells. Peyer's patches showed lymphoid hyperplasia with an increase of mononuclear cells. The livers were grossly normal. Microscopically they showed abscesses, congestion, and focal necrosis. Kupffer's cells contained bacteria. The spleens also were congested with lymphoid hyperplasia of the white pulp and necrosis in the red pulp. Large numbers of bacteria were visible in the liver sinusoids and red pulp of the spleens. Examination of the mesenteric lymph nodes revealed lymphoid hyperplasia without necrosis or abscess formation. In most animals there were increased numbers of mononuclear cells with phagocytic activity (Figure 5.1).

To observe the sequential appearance of pathological changes, other groups of mice were sacrificed at 6, 12, 24, 48, and 72 hr after intragastric inoculation with 8×10^5 organisms. No pathologic changes were noted in the first 12 hr, but changes became apparent 24 hr after the infection. In the gastrointestinal tract, the overlying intestinal mucosa was intact throughout. Peyer's patches contained mononuclear cells with phagocytosed nuclear debris, and the number of mononuclear cells increased with time. In the liver and spleen, organisms were present in the sinusoidal spaces and were engulfed by the reticuloendothelial lining cells at 24 hr. Microabscesses containing bacteria were evident at 48 hr and extensive necrosis was noted at 72 hr. The mesenteric lymph nodes were hyperplastic with increased numbers of mononuclear cells in the sinuses. Some of the mononuclear cells contained bacterial organisms at 72 hr. No pathology was found in the lungs, kidney, or pancreas. Bacteria were, however, found in the blood vessels of all organs.

To determine whether the observed changes in intestinal epithelium, Peyer's patches, and mesenteric lymph nodes were attributable to the introduction of organisms into the gastrointestinal tract, these tissues were compared between groups of mice inoculated by the intragastric and subcutaneous routes. Both groups showed comparable, similar changes. This identical pathology in infections that were introduced by both routes indicated that the lesions of orally induced plague infections were probably the result of systemic infection rather than of local enteric infection.

To assess the ability of *Y. pestis* to survive the acid pH of the stomach

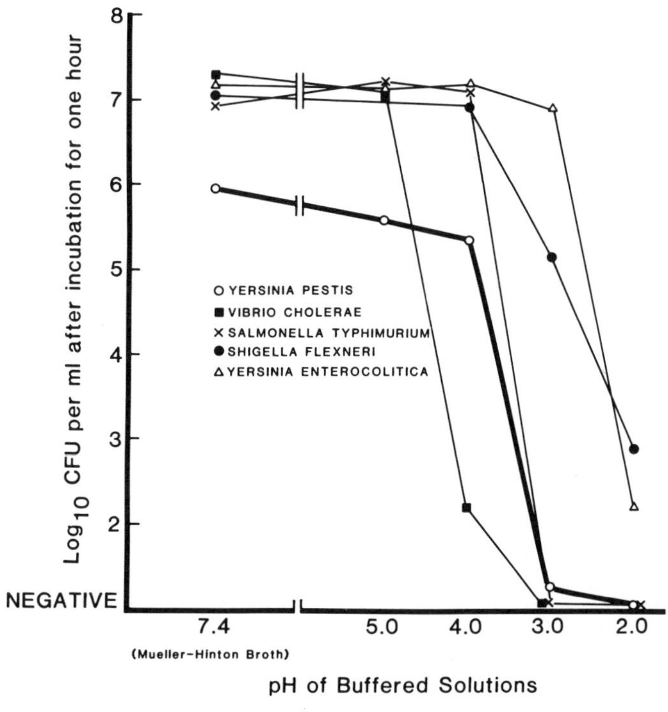

FIGURE 5.2. Antibacterial effect of acidity on suspensions of *Y. pestis* (Vietnam). Each point is the mean of triplicate plate counts determining the colony-forming units (CFU) of bacteria after 1 hr of incubation at 37°C in citrate–phosphate buffers of given pHs. Results of cultures of *Vibrio cholerae, Salmonella typhimurium, Y. enterocolitica,* and *Shigella flexneri* are also shown.

following ingestion or intragastric inoculation, we placed one part log-phase cultures in Mueller–Hinton broth into nine parts of sodium diphosphate–citric acid buffers at different pH values. After 1 hr of incubation at 37°C, viable bacteria were counted. As shown in Figure 5.2, one strain of *Y. pestis* isolated from a patient in Vietnam survived pH values of 4 and higher, but was sharply killed at pH values of 3 and lower. This pattern was similar to the LT-2 strain of *Salmonella typhimurium*. When compared to other species of bacteria, *Y. pestis* was more resistant to acid pH than *Vibrio cholerae*, but was more sensitive than tested strains of *Y. enterocolitica* and *Shigella flexneri*.

To elucidate the sequence of bacterial proliferation in different tissues, quantitative cultures of homogenized organs and tissues were obtained 6 hr, 12 hr, 24 hr, and 48 hr after intragastric challenge with 3×10^8 viable organisms. As shown in Table 5.7, bacteria accumulated to levels greater than $\log_2$ per tissue at 12 hr in the spleen, liver, and blood. In these tissues the numbers of bacteria continued to accumulate until 48 hr. In the intestinal lymphoid tissue of Peyer's patches and mesenteric lymph nodes, bacteria appeared in smaller quantities and more slowly than in the spleen, liver, and blood. Only at 48 hr had the mesenteric lymph nodes acquired more than $\log_4$ bacteria per node. This level of infection had been reached in the spleen and liver as early as 12 hr after inoculation. These findings indicated that *Y. pestis* infection by the oral route bypasses intestinal tissues by proceeding directly to become a systemic infection of the blood, spleen, and liver (Table 5.7).

TABLE 5.7
Progression of Infection through Tissues of CF-1 Mice Inoculated Intragastrically with a Suspension of 3×10^8 Viable *Yersinia pestis* in 0.2 ml of 0.9% NaCl

	Mean ± S.E.M. $\log_{10}$ CFU *Y. pestis* in tissues[a]				
Hours after inoculation	Peyer's patches	Mesenteric lymph node	Spleen	Liver	Blood
6	None	None	0.89 ± 0.19	None	None
12	0.77 ± 0.08	0.80 ± 0.19	4.09 ± 0.39	4.91 ± 0.44	2.49 ± 0.77
24	1.21 ± 0.30	2.21 ± 0.51	3.86 ± 1.12	4.93 ± 1.42	3.60 ± 0.99
48	0.89 ± 0.19	4.94 ± 0.47	5.83 ± 0.49	7.02 ± 0.42	4.95 ± 0.43

[a] For Peyer's patches, mesenteric lymph nodes, and spleen, each number is the mean ± S.E.M. of the $\log_{10}$ CFU (colony-forming units) of *Y. pestis* per total tissue obtained in each of four mice. For liver and blood, results are the mean ± S.E.M. of the $\log_{10}$ CFU of *Y. pestis* per gram of tissue obtained in each of four mice. The limit of detectability was 10 bacteria per tissue. Negative cultures were counted as five bacteria, or $\log_{10}$ = 0.70. None indicates all specimens showed negative cultures.

After intragastric challenges with doses containing as many as 10^9 *Y. pestis* organisms, stools were collected daily for 3 days from 25 mice and from 10 rats. Stools were emulsified in saline, serially diluted, and plated onto trypticase soy agar and deoxycholate agar. All stool cultures were negative for *Y. pestis*. To determine how well inoculated *Y. pestis* survives in the intestine, five mice were killed 1 hr after intragastric challenge with 3×10^8 organisms. The stomach and small bowel were flushed with saline. These effluents also gave negative cultures for *Y. pestis,* indicating that bacteria did not survive in the lumen of the stomach and bowel.

In experiments to determine the LD50 and ID50 values of *Y. pestis* by intragastric challenge, rodents that survived for 21 days or longer were killed and serum obtained for measurement of antibodies against Fraction IA of *Y. pestis*. Most animals that received the larger doses died before the time of serological testing. As shown in Table 5.8, 6 of 57 surviving mice, or 11% showed increased titers of antibody. All 57 had negative spleen cultures at this time, indicating that the six with elevated antibody titers had developed self-limited infections. None of eight tested *Z. pixuna* had antibody elevations; the smaller number available for testing resulted from the high mortality rate in this group, indicating that they were susceptible to lethal infection but not to self-limited infection. *R. rattus* showed a higher rate of serological responses, 8 of 15 or 53%, that was associated with larger LD50 and ID50 values, indicating that the rats were relatively resistant to developing infection but that some did develop self-limited infection (Table 5.8).

These results showed that *Y. pestis* was an effective oral pathogen by producing fatal systemic infections and self-limited infections with immunity, but that it did not produce enteric pathology or lead to fecal excretion of

TABLE 5.8
Immune Response in Rodents Surviving Intragastric Inoculation of Virulent *Yersinia pestis*

Species of rodent	Dose (range of inoculated viable bacteria)	No. of rodents with elevated PHA titers/total survivors[a]
M. musculus	1.1×10^2–1.1×10^7	6/57
Z. pixuna	1.7×10^4–1.7×10^9	0/8
R. rattus	4.2×10^5–4.2×10^9	8/15

[a] (PHA) Passive hemagglutination.

bacteria. This suggests that rodents may acquire infection in nature by eating other dead animals or ingesting other materials contaminated with remains of dead animals in soil. Although the infective doses of *Y. pestis* by the oral route were higher than by the subcutaneous route, the large numbers of bacteria in the tissues of dying animals would provide ample inocula for infection to occur by the oral route.

5.2. *YERSINIA ENTEROCOLITICA* INFECTION

The experimental studies of the pathogenesis of *Y. enterocolitica* infections indicate that infection with this species differs sharply from *Y. pestis* by producing localized invasive infection in the intestine and by eliciting diarrhea in the host. In this section, I will summarize selected recent work dealing with experimental animal infections, mechanisms of invasion, virulence antigens, plasmids, and enterotoxin production by *Y. enterocolitica*. Considerable amounts of work have been carried out by investigators on *Y. enterocolitica* during the past decade. The Third International Symposium on *Yersinia* Infections was held in Montreal, Canada, in 1977. The proceedings of that Symposium were published in 1980,[48b] and the reader is referred to this publication for more detailed information on these infections.

5.2.1. Experimental Infections

5.2.1.1. Rodents

Earlier work by Mollaret and Guillon in 1965[(49)] failed to reveal virulence of 106 strains of *Y. enterocolitica* in rodents. These strains belonged to serotypes O:3 and O:9. This lack of virulence may have been related to strain differences, because certain serotypes such as O:8 have been shown to be highly virulent in rodents. Subsequently, Nilehn[(50)] showed that mice were susceptible to lethal infections with certain strains of serotypes O:3 and O:9 when large doses of bacteria, in the range of 10^8–10^9 organisms, were given by the intraperitoneal route. Bacteria grown at 25°C were more lethal than bacteria grown at 37°C, and these bacteria grown at 25°C were shown to persist longer in the peritoneal cavity of the mouse.

In 1974 Quan *et al.*[(51)] reported that two strains of *Y. entercolitica* isolated from human sources belonging to serotypes O:8 and O:4 killed mice after subcutaneous injection with about 10^4 organisms. At autopsy the mice showed large nodular lesions in the spleen and liver and caseous masses at the site of inoculation. Intraperitoneal inoculation gave an LD50 that was 1000-fold less than that by subcutaneous inoculation.

Carter and co-workers[(52–54)] demonstrated that a human isolate of serotype O:8 was pathogenic in laboratory mice. An intragastric inoculation of 5×10^7 organisms infected animals and produced an enteric infection that progressed stepwise through Peyer's patches, mesenteric lymph nodes, liver, and spleen. In less than 24 hr after inoculation mice showed neutrophilic infiltration of Peyer's patches of the distal ileum, and abscesses formed also in the mesenteric lymph nodes. The abscesses in Peyer's patches progressed to ulceration of the adjacent ileal mucosa and sometimes to perforation of the intestine with resultant peritonitis. Rapid multiplication of organisms followed with dissemination to liver, spleen, and lungs, resulting in a fatal outcome. When this strain of *Y. enterocolitica* was administered by the intravenous route, a dose of only 500 organisms was lethal. When given by an aerogenic challenge 1000 organisms produced fatal pneumonia. Cultivation of this strain at 25°C before inoculation resulted in faster multiplication of bacteria in the spleen and liver and a slower clearance from blood when compared to cultivation of bacteria at 37°C. This greater virulence of bacteria grown at 25°C was related to resistance of organisms to intracellular killing after phagocytosis.

The cause of death in mice infected with *Y. enterocolitica* was also studied by Carter.[(52)] He estimated that fatal infections were produced after bacteria had reached a quantity of at least 10^9 bacteria per mouse. The lethal dose of whole killed bacteria was about 10^{10} organisms or 2200 μg of bacteria. This lethality of a large quantity of whole bacteria produced by experimental injections of whole bacteria, as well as the presence of a large mass of bacteria at the time of death during the course of experimental infection, is similar to bacteriological findings in plague infection and suggested that the endotoxin of *Y. enterocolitica* may play a role in pathogenicity.

Although serotypes O:3 and O:9 were shown to be relatively nonlethal for mice, Ricciardi *et al.*[(55)] showed that intraperitoneal inoculation of these strains into mice resulted in long-term fecal excretion. This fecal excretion was constant and lasted for as long as 135 days. Although the infections were nonfatal, protective immunity developed, as shown by a reduced mortality when mice were rechallenged with 500 LD50s 35 days after the original infection. Thus, certain strains of *Y. enterocolitica* appear to be well adapted to rodents, and this suggests that rodents could be reservoirs of infection in nature by tolerating the infection and remaining chronic excreters of bacteria.

Mongolian gerbils were shown to be more susceptible to experimental *Y. enterocolitica* infections than were mice. Quan *et al.*[51] showed that as few as 250 bacteria injected intraperitoneally killed the gerbil. One strain of serotype O:8 that was examined by Schiemann and Devenish[56] killed gerbils after injection of only 100 bacteria intraperitoneally. Gerbils were also susceptible to fatal infections when inoculated orally by a feeding tube with 10^6 to 10^7 organisms.

The lack of virulence of serotypes O:3 and O:9 in some experimental rodent infections led to attempts to immunosuppress animals. A variety of manipulations, including use of germ-free animals, use of athymic nude mice, irradiation, and treatments with cyclophosphamide or ferrous ammonium citrate, have been employed by workers to increase the susceptibility of laboratory animals to *Y. enterocolitica* infection. Bazin *et al.*[57] exposed rats to 5.7 Gray doses of whole-body irradiation and 5 or 10 days later injected them intravenously with 10^8 organisms of *Y. enterocolitica* serotype O:3. These rats showed an increased death rate, but no increased susceptibility was observed when bacteria were given by the oral route. Athymic nude mice, B-lymphocyte-depleted mice, and macrophage-deficient mice were not more susceptible to this bacterial strain. These workers concluded that irradiation enhanced susceptibility to lethal infection by altering systemic host defenses by a mechanism other than that of the T- or B-lymphocyte-dependent immune system.

Another successful approach to enhance the virulence of *Y. enterocolitica* in rodents is to give iron to animals. Robins-Browne *et al.*[58] administered 200 μg of ferrous ammonium citrate intraperitoneally to mice 24 hr before 10^9 organisms of *Y. enterocolitica* serotype O:3 were given by the same route. The mortality rate of these mice was enhanced, and the postmortem pathology showed abscesses and necrosis in the liver and deposition of fibrin in blood vessels, suggesting a pathological process of endotoxemia. In similar experiments, Smith *et al.*[59] injected mice intraperitoneally with 0.5 cm^3 of 20% iron–dextran at the same time as *Y. enterocolitica* organisms of serotypes O:3 and O:9. Lethality of infected mice was increased over the control mice, and the iron–dextran enabled the bacteria to cause internal liver lesions. The mechanism of the iron-induced enhancement of infection was not established in these experiments. The two possible interpretations were that iron acted on the bacteria to increase the growth rate and that iron interfered with normal host defense mechanisms. The latter possibility was examined by Robins-Browne *et al.*[58] in an experiment with normal human serum that was bactericidal against the O:3 serotype of *Y. enterocolitica*. Addition of ferrous ammonium citrate to the serum in an amount sufficient to saturate transferrin abolished the serum bactericidal activity. Thus, the mechanism of iron-induced enhancement of infection is likely to be, in part, neutralization of host antibacterial defenses.

5.2.1.2. Rabbits

White laboratory rabbits have been demonstrated to be useful animal models for intestinal infection and development of diarrhea. Une[60] inoculated an isolate of *Y. enterocolitica* serotype O:3 obtained from a patient in Japan into white rabbits by intraduodenal injection during laparotomy. Two to three days after inoculation with 10^7–10^9 organisms, rabbits developed diarrhea and stool cultures were positive for the organism for as long as 40 days. Organisms could also be recovered from mesenteric lymph nodes, liver, and spleen. Pathological examination revealed ulceration of the intestine associated with bacterial penetration of the lamina propria with bacterial multiplication. The inflammatory cells were predominantly mononuclear with some neutrophils. Bacteria were seen within mononuclear phagocytes. Granulomas were observed in lymph follicles of lymph nodes, liver, and spleen.

The rabbit was also used by Pai *et al.*[61] to inoculate a Canadian strain of serotype O:3. They used young New Zealand white rabbits (weighing between 500 and 800 g), which received inocula by orogastric feeding. The ID50 was 2.9×10^8 bacteria with the appearance of diarrhea after 5 days. Thirty percent of the rabbits that received more than 10^{10} bacteria died. Bacterial excretion in stools occurred in all rabbits with and without diarrhea, starting 1 day after inoculation and continuing for as long as 3 weeks. Pathology consisted of crypt abscesses that occurred predominantly in the ileum but also in the jejunum and colon. The abscesses were comprised of bacteria, neutrophils, eosinophils, and mononuclear cells. The adjacent crypt epithelium was focally necrotic and ulcerated. Lymphoid tissue was hyperplastic. Bacteria were also isolated from the liver and spleen, indicating that dissemination of infection from the crypt abscesses had occurred. This rabbit model is, thus, useful both for the study of the local intestinal disease leading to diarrhea and for the systemic features of fatal disease with dissemination of bacteria to liver and spleen.

5.2.2. Invasive Properties of *Yersinia enterocolitica*

The ability of virulent strains to penetrate host cells is a necessary feature for virulence. *In vitro* tests of invasiveness have been demonstrated to be positive for human isolates of *Y. enterocolitica*. Mäki *et al.*[(62)] showed that 21 of 24 strains invaded cultured human epithelial cells. Some of these strains had been isolated from diarrheal patients who had shown polymorphonuclear leukocytes in the stool, indicating that the bacteria had caused clinically invasive enteritis. Similarly, Une[(63)] showed that strains of *Y. enterocolitica* of serotypes O:3 and O:9 isolated from patients in Japan penetrated HeLa cells. Furthermore, he showed that these strains were phagocytosed by rabbit peritoneal macrophages and that bacteria survived intracellularly after phagocytosis.

Another test for bacterial invasiveness is the inducement of conjunctivitis in guinea pigs, called the Sereny test. It has been widely used to show the invasiveness of *Shigella* strains and enteroinvasive strains of *E. coli*. Schiemann and Devenish showed that human isolates of serotype O:8 were positive in Sereny tests but that human strains of serotype O:3 were negative.[(56)] Thus, some but not all invasive strains show positive reactions in the Sereny test, and this test cannot be used as a sole criterion for virulence. Mors and Pai[(64)] have suggested that HeLa-cell invasiveness is consistently found in several different human pathogenic serotypes.

A recently recognized virulence determinant of *Y. enterocolitica* is the VW antigen complex, which is also present in virulent strains of *Y. pestis* and *Y. pseudotuberculosis*. The V and W antigens have been detected in *Y. enterocolitica* by Schiemann and Devenish[(56)] and by Gemski *et al.*[(65)] through the demonstration of failure to grow in a calcium-deficient medium at 37°C. Avirulent strains, on the other hand, will grow in the calcium-deficient medium.

5.2.3. Plasmid-Mediated Control of Invasiveness

Zink *et al.*[(66)] examined a human isolate of serotype O:8 from the United States. Using agarose gel electrophoresis, they found plasmid DNA in all virulent strains. The molecular weights of the plasmid DNA were 41×10^6 and 35×10^6. All strains that were invasive by the Sereny test contained the

41×10^6 mol. wt. plasmid. Removal of plasmid DNA by ethidium bromide treatment caused a loss of invasiveness. One strain retained only the 35×10^6 mol. wt. plasmid, and it was not invasive. Thus, the 41×10^6 mol. wt. plasmid appeared to control invasiveness of *Y. enterocolitica* in this study. Gemski *et al.*[(65)] confirmed that a plasmid of similar molecular weight, 42×10^6, was associated with tissue invasiveness in strains of serotype O:8. Furthermore, they showed that the same plasmid was associated with the VW antigen complex. Bacterial colonies that grew in the absence of calcium were shown to have lost the plasmid and the ability to cause a positive Sereny test. J. Heesemann *et al.*[66a] showed that human strains of serotypes O:3 and O:9 harbored plasmids of 46 and 44 megadaltons, respectively, and that these plasmids encoded properties of calcium dependence, survival in 25–75% human serum, and positive Sereny tests.

A new plasmid with a molecular weight of 82 megadaltons was described by Kay *et al.*[(67)] This plasmid confers the property of lethality to mice. Serotypes other than O:3 and O:9 were shown to harbor this plasmid, and some of these serotypes were isolated from the environment and have been considered nonpathogenic for humans (Table 5.9).

TABLE 5.9
Plasmids of *Yersinia enterocolitica* Controlling Virulence

Virulence factor	Serotype(s)	Plasmid characteristic mol. wt. in megadaltons
Autoagglutination	O:3	46
	O:8	
V W antigens and calcium dependency	O:3	41, 42
	O:9	
Tissue invasive (Sereny test)	O:8	41, 42
Lethality for mice	O:8	82
	O:40	
	O:20	
	O:13	
Survival in human serum	O:3	46
	O:9	44

5.2.4. Enterotoxin Production by *Yersinia enterocolitica*

Pathogenic strains of *Y. enterocolitica* have been shown to elaborate an enterotoxin, which may explain the mechanism of diarrhea in patients with *Yersinia* gastroenteritis.[(68)] The enterotoxin is produced in cultures of bacteria and can be detected in the supernatants after bacteria are removed by centrifugation. This enterotoxin was shown to be produced only at lower incubation temperature of 25°C but not at 37°C. Enterotoxin activity was assayed either by the infant mouse test or in rabbit ileal loops.[(69)] Negative results were obtained using the Y1 adrenal cell assay, which detects cholera toxin and *E. coli* heat-labile toxin.[(69)]

Boyce and co-workers[(70)] showed that the enterotoxin of *Y. enterocolitica* resembled the heat-stable enterotoxin (ST) of *E. coli* by demonstrating that it retained activity after being heated to 121°C. They showed further that it resisted acidity down to pH 1 and was soluble in methanol. Another similarity of *Y. enterocolitica* enterotoxin to *E. coli* ST was demonstrated by Robins-Browne *et al.*,[(69)] who showed that the enterotoxin of *Y. enterocolitica* activated the enzyme guanylate cyclase in the infant mouse intestine, but did not activate adenylate cyclase. Rao *et al.*[(71)] confirmed these results by showing that intestinal cell membranes contained increased amounts of cyclic guanosine 3′,5′-monophosphate after exposure to the toxin. Further, they demonstrated that this toxin produced diarrhea by increasing the short-circuit current of rabbit distal ileum in an Ussing chamber and also inhibited active chloride absorption across the short-circuited ileal mucosa.

The chemical and immunological nature of the enterotoxin has been characterized by Okamoto and co-workers.[(72)] By methods of column chromatography, gel filtration, and isoelectric focusing, they showed that the enterotoxin of *Y. enterocolitica* is a protein with a molecular weight of about 9000. Two toxic components, ST-1 and ST-2, could be separated by isoelectric focusing. Enterotoxic activity was not removed by treatment with trypsin, protease, lipase, phospholipase C, ribonuclease, deoxyribonuclease, β-glucosidase, and neuraminidase. Antiserum prepared by immunizing guinea pigs with toxin from *Y. enterocolitica* neutralized both the homologous enterotoxin and ST of *E. coli*. This immunological cross-reactivity demonstrated a further structural similarity between the active toxic sites of the molecules of *E. coli* ST and the enterotoxin of *Y. enterocolitica*.

Despite these several similarities between *E. coli* ST and the enterotoxin of *Y. enterocolitica*, there are also some important differences (Table 5.10).

TABLE 5.10
Comparison of the Heat-Stable Enterotoxin (ST) of *Escherichia coli* to the Enterotoxin of *Yersinia enterocolitica*

	E. coli ST	*Y. enterocolitica* enterotoxin
Optimal temperature for production of cultures	37°C	25°C
Phase of bacterial growth at which toxin is produced	Early logarithmic	Late stationary
Genetic control	Plasmid mediated	Chromosomal
Molecular weight	4400	9000
Effective dose in infant mouse assay	14 ng	110 ng
Heat stability	Stable at 100°C, destroyed at 121°C	Stable at 121°C

The enterotoxin of *Y. enterocolitica* is produced only at lower temperatures of 25°C and is produced even at refrigeration temperatures of 3–6°C.[(73)] Boyce was able to detect enterotoxin in cultures of *Y. enterocolitica* only in the late stationary phase of growth when the available glucose in the media had been consumed, whereas *E. coli* ST is produced in early logarithmic growth. Zink *et al.*[(66)] showed that strains of pathogenic *Y. enterocolitica* that had lost the plasmid-controlling invasiveness retained their toxin-producing capacity. Finally, the molecular weights and effective doses of the two toxins are different.[(74,75)]

Although the enterotoxin production by *Y. enterocolitica* can be viewed as a basis for diarrheal pathogenicity, considerable doubt has been cast on the actual relevance of the enterotoxin in human disease. The failure of the enterotoxin to be produced at the human body temperature of 37°C makes it unlikely that enterotoxin would be elaborated in infected tissues to lead to diarrhea. Furthermore, the enterotoxin is not produced under anaerobic conditions that prevail in the intestinal lumen where the presumed enterotoxin should be elaborated. Thus, it appears that, as with other invasive intestinal pathogens such as *Shigella* species, the primary determinant of virulence is tissue invasiveness and that the enterotoxin is a marker of the bacterium which does not have an established role in pathogenicity.

Despite the demonstration of tissue invasiveness and enterotoxin production in pathogenic strains of *Y. enterocolitica,* the pathogenesis of diarrhea has not been fully explained. We do not know why children are more susceptible to the diarrheal manifestations and older children and adults are more prone to have ileitis or mesenteric adenitis without diarrhea. Other forms of diarrhea, similarly, affect children more acutely than adults. For example, children with shigellosis have a tendency to present with watery diarrhea and adults present with dysentery.[76] Typhoid fever is also commonly a diarrheal disease in children but not often in adults.[77]

The typical pathology of localized ileitis and mesenteric lymphadenitis, often with fever, in *Y. enterocolitica* infection suggests that other, unrecognized, mechanisms may play a role in the pathogenesis of diarrhea. With an organism that has a predilection to invade only the terminal ileum, it seems unlikely that an adequate quantity of the heat-stable enterotoxin could be produced and delivered to the small intestinal mucosa, the presumed site of enterotoxin action. It appears more plausible that there is systemic mediation of the diarrhea that is a part of the host response to invasive infection. This kind of "parenteral diarrhea," has been proposed to explain diarrhea that accompanies acute infections, such as pneumonia, that do not directly involve the intestine.

5.2.5. Role of Serum Complement and Bacterial Endotoxin in Pathogenesis

Nilehn[50] showed that normal human serum was bactericidal against human strains of *Y. enterocolitica*. She showed additionally that when bacteria were grown at 37°C they were more susceptible to the bactericidal action of serum than when bacteria were grown at 25°C. The role of complement in the killing of *Yersinia* was further studied by Acker and Brade.[78] They showed that a strain of *Y. enterocolitica* was killed completely by incubation in 30% human serum. Removal of lysozyme did not diminish killing, but heating the serum at 56°C for 30 min abolished the killing, indicating that the complement system was involved in the bactericidal effect. Treatment of serum with magnesium-ethyleneglycol-tetraacetic acid (Mg-EGTA) to inactivate the classical complement pathway reduced the killing, but addition of further Mg-EGTA-treated serum restored full bactericidal action, indicating that the alternative complement pathway, as well as the classical pathway, was active in killing this strain of *Y. enterocolitica*. By electron microscopy serum was shown to cause destruction of the murine layer of the cell wall with the production of blebs and cell envelope fragments. Acker and Brade[78] demonstrated also that serum in which bacteria had been incubated showed a loss of complement activity and that the complement protein C3b was deposited on the bacterial surface. Because phagocytic cells contain receptors on their surfaces for C3b, this finding suggests that serum can render *Y. enterocolitica* susceptible to phagocytosis.

These findings suggest that complement proteins may play roles in both host defenses against disseminated infection and the expression of disease in the host. The ability of normal serum to kill *Y. enterocolitica* means that bacteria cannot survive long in the blood or other serum-containing spaces of the body. Thus, infection is likely to be localized to intracellular environments such as the lymphoid tissue of the intestine. Bacteremia should be rare, and bacteria should not be able to multiply in the blood and reach fatal densities, as may occur in plague infection. The possibility that serum-resistant strains of *Y. enterocolitica* may be associated with cases of bacteremic infection has not been explored. On the other hand, Pai and De Stephano[79] examined a virulent strain of serotype O:3 and found it to be resistant to serum killing in 10% human serum. A derivative of this strain that was avirulent in rabbits and had lost properties of autoagglutination and calcium dependency was shown to be susceptible to serum killing. The disparity between the findings of these workers could be caused by bacterial strain differences or the concentrations of serum used. It seems logical, however, that invasive bacteria must possess at least some degree of resistance to serum killing in order to be effective pathogens in animal tissues.

The deposition of C3b on the surface of *Y. enterocolitica* would assist host phagocytes to make necessary contact with bacteria and to engulf them for intracellular killing. The expression of disease may be, in part, mediated by complement proteins. The activation of the complement system results in several active products, such as C5a, a mediator of anaphylaxis, and vasoactive substances which may lower blood pressure.

The interaction of *Y. enterocolitica* with serum proteins involves LPS. Brade and Kreuzpaintner[80] demonstrated that LPS of *Y. enterocolitica,* like LPS from other gram-negative bacteria, contains Lipid A and may be either from smooth colonies with a complete O-side chain or from rough colonies with incomplete O-side chains. They showed that rough LPS binds directly to serum C3, thus activating complement proteins. Lipid A and smooth LPS were more efficient in activating complement in whole serum. From other studies that have differentiated the two major complement pathways, it can be concluded that Lipid A predominantly activates the classical pathway and the polysaccharides of the O-side chains of smooth LPS activate the alternative pathway.

Structural studies of the O-side chains of the LPS of *Y. enterocolitica* (YE 128) have been carried out by Hoffman *et al.*[81] They showed that the O-antigen is a homopolymer composed of (1 → 2)-linked 6-deoxy-β-L-altro-pyranosyl residues and that they are linked in a $^{1}C_4$ conformation.

5.2.6. Temperature Dependence of Virulence of *Yersinia enterocolitica*

Whereas *Y. pestis* is more virulent when grown at 37°C than at lower ambient temperatures that exist outside the infected host, *Y. enterocolitica* appears to exhibit the opposite pattern of showing greater virulence when grown at 25°C than at 37°C. The greater virulence at 25°C was shown by Nilehn[50] to be related to greater resistance to the serum bactericidal action and resistance to phagocytic killing. Furthermore, Nilehn showed that bacteria grown at 25°C have two or more peritrichous flagellae, but that these flagellae are lost in cultures grown at 37°C.[82] Zink *et al.*[66] showed further that cultivation of bacteria at 37°C resulted in loss of the 41×10^6 mol.wt. plasmid and loss of invasiveness. On the other hand, Pai and De Stephano showed that serum resistance in virulent strains of *Y. enterocolitica* was expressed during growth at 37°C but not at 25°C.[79] Other properties of autoagglutination and calcium dependence were also lost during growth at 25°C.

Thus, it appears that *Y. enterocolitica* at lower temperatures in the environment, as would be found after passage of organisms in the stool, acquires certain properties of motility and resistance to phagocytic defenses that allow bacteria to invade. After the bacteria have become established in the host, these properties of virulence are temporarily lost. Perhaps at this later time, after growth of 37°C, certain other properties, such as serum resistance, are acquired and allow bacteria sometimes to disseminate from the initial focus of infection in the intestine and its lymphoid tissue.

5.2.7. Role of Iron in Pathogenesis

Like the other yersiniae, *Y. enterocolitica* cannot synthesize its own iron-binding compounds called siderophores (or chromatophores). Other pathogenic bacteria, including *Salmonella* and *Shigella* species, can synthesize siderophores which are considered virulence factors.[83,84] Because iron is necessary for bacterial growth and exists in low growth-limiting concentrations in animal tissues, the yersiniae must acquire iron-binding siderophores from other bacteria or from host tissues. It has been previously noted that patients with excessive tissue iron, as occurs in hemochromatosis, are predisposed to disseminated *Yersinia* infections. Furthermore, the treatment of animals with iron salts renders them more susceptible to experimental infection with *Yersinia*.

One of the most direct connections between iron treatment and the appearance of disseminated *Y. enterocolitica* was reported from Norway by Melby *et al.*[85] Two children took oral overdoses of ferrocarbonate and ferrous fumarate. To counteract the overdoses, both received the iron-chelating drug desferrioxamine. Within 1 day after ingesting the iron, both children developed fever and had *Y. enterocolitica* isolated from blood cultures. It must be considered that the iron gave the bacteria a growth advantage. Another possibility is that the iron-chelator desferrioxamine was used by the bacteria as a siderophore; it is known that *Y. enterocolitica* grows better in the presence of this compound. Still another explanation for this striking association between iron and *Yersinia* septicemia was that the iron salts damaged the intestinal epithelium, allowing bacteria to enter the circulation. Additionally, the demonstration by Robins-Browne *et al.*[58] that iron ions can neutralize bactericidal activity of human serum indicates that iron may have acted on host defenses after bacterial invasion.

5.2.8. Pathogenesis of *Yersinia* Arthritis

The complication of arthritis that has been frequently reported from Scandinavian countries has been termed reactive arthritis because bacteria cannot usually be recovered from the affected joints. A strong association between individuals with the genotype HLA-B27 has been documented. HLA-B27 is a gene product of one of the alleles of the major histocompatibility complex and predisposes persons to many other forms of reactive arthritis, such as Reiter's syndrome. In Finland, Leirisalo *et al.*[86] studied polymorphonuclear leukocyte motility in persons with *Y. enterocolitica* infection and in controls, some of whom had HLA-B27. They showed that leukocytes from HLA-B27-positive individuals showed greater chemotactic activity in response to zymosan-activated serum than leukocytes from HLA-B27-negative persons. This greater chemotactic activity of the polymorphonuclear leukocytes in HLA-B27-positive individuals provides an explanation for the marked predisposition of persons with HLA-B27 to develop arthritis after *Yersinia* infection.

5.3. *YERSINIA PSEUDOTUBERCULOSIS* INFECTION

Owing to the rarity of recognized *Y. pseudotuberculosis* infections in humans, less research has been carried out with this organism. There are many similarities between it and *Y. enterocolitica,* and much of the information obtained for *Y. enterocolitica* infections may be applicable. Both organisms produce enteric infections with a predilection for the intestinal lymphoid tissue. Disseminated infections occur in patients with liver diseases or with other immunocompromises. *Y. pseudotuberculosis* is not, however, a recognized cause of diarrhea as *Y. enterocolitica* has come to be. In this section, I will discuss some selected work relating to the pathogenesis of *Y. pseudotuberculosis*.

5.3.1. Experimental Infections

Une[87] injected 10^8 organisms of a human strain of *Y. pseudotuberculosis* intraduodenally into rabbits. All inoculated rabbits developed diarrhea within 2–3 days and died within 8 days, whereas the same inoculum size of *Y. enterocolitica* was not fatal to the rabbits. More than 10^7 bacteria/g of tissue were recovered from the mesenteric lymph nodes, liver, and spleen. The small intestine showed petechial hemorrhages and miliary white patches on the serosal surface. Microscopically, there were mucosal ulcerations in the ileum. The lamina propria showed a mononuclear infiltrate. In the lymphoid follicles of the intestine, mesenteric lymph nodes, liver, and spleen, there were well-developed granulomas with necrotic centers. Bacteria were concentrated in the necrotic centers of the granulomas.

5.3.2. Invasiveness for HeLa Cells

Bovallius and Nilsson[88] showed that a strain of *Y. pseudotuberculosis* of O-antigen group I penetrated HeLa cells in *in vitro* culture. After a lag time of about 1 hr, penetration was rapid and occurred in a manner that resembled phagocytosis. Electron microscopy documented a membrane contact, invagination of the membrane, engulfment, and formation of phagocytic vacuoles. Intracellular bacteria survived for at least 3 days. Une[87] confirmed the infectivity of Japanese strains of *Y. pseudotuberculosis* for HeLa cells.

5.3.3. Lipopolysaccharides of *Yersinia pseudotuberculosis*

Like other gram-negative bacteria belonging to the family Enterobacteriaceae, *Y. pseudotuberculosis* possesses LPS as a structural component of its cell wall. The LPS has O-specific polysaccharide side chains that differ from those of other bacterial species. Samuelsson and co-workers[89] analyzed chemically these O-specific side chains from 10 different serotypes of *Y. pseudotuberculosis*. They found all five of the 3,6-dideoxyhexoses that are known to occur in nature. Furthermore, the sugar 6-deoxy-D-manno-heptose was found in some serotypes and this sugar is not known to occur elsewhere in nature. Gorshkova *et al.*[90] carried out structural studies on the O-specific polysaccharides of *Y. pseudotuberculosis,* type III. They found equimolar quantities of the four sugars paratose, L-fucose, D-mannose, and 2-deoxy-2-amino-D-galactose. They suggested that there is a repeating unit of these four sugars in the polysaccharide.

5.3.4. Other Virulence Determinants of *Yersinia pseudotuberculosis*

Brubaker[91] has pointed out that *Y. pseudotuberculosis* may be a less invasive bacterium than *Y. pestis* because the former lacks the coagulase and fibrinolysin enzymes that are properties of *Y. pestis*. In certain other respects, the two organisms are similar. Both possess the VW antigen complex, which is synthesized by bacteria incubated under aerobic conditions at 37°C in the absence of calcium and in the presence of magnesium ions. These conditions approximate the intracellular environment of mammalian cells. Bacteria possessing the VW antigen complex do not multiply rapidly in this calcium-free environment but express the VW antigen complex. When calcium is added to a culture, bacteria grow faster and cease to express the VW antigen complex. Brubaker showed that the VW antigen complex was associated with virulence by demonstrating that the LD50 for mice after intravenous injection was about 40 bacteria of a strain with the VW antigen complex and greater than 10^8 bacteria of a strain lacking the VW antigen complex. Because the VW antigen complex is expressed under conditions that resemble the intracellular environment, these virulence antigens may permit bacteria to survive and multiply within cells. The ability of bacteria with the VW antigen complex to multiply in the greater ionic strength with high potassium concentrations and low sodium concentrations within cells is a suggested mechanism for the virulence produced by this antigen.

REFERENCES

1. R. R. Brubaker, Expression of virulence in yersiniae, in *Microbiology—1979* (D. Schlessinger, ed.), American Society for Microbiology, Washington (1979).
2. R. R. Brukaer, The genus *Yersinia:* Biochemistry and genetics of virulence, *Curr. Top. Microbiol. Immunol.* **57:**111–158 (1972).
3. R. V. Walker, Plague toxins: A critical review, *Curr. Top. Microbiol. Immunol.* **41:**23–60 (1967).
4. T. C. Montie and S. J. Ajl, Nature and synthesis of murine toxins of *Pasteurella pestis,* in *Microbial Toxins,* Volume 3 (T. C. Montie, S. Kadis, and S. J. Ajl, eds.), Academic Press, New York, (1970).
5. T. C. Montie, D. B. Montie, and D. Wennerstrom, Aspects of structure and biological activity of plague murine toxin, in *Microbiology—1975* (D. Schlessinger, ed.), American Society for Microbiology, Washington (1975).
6. T. C. Montie, Properties and pharmacological action of plague murine toxin, *Pharmacol. Ther.* **12:**491–499 (1981).
7. R. Glosnicka and E. Gruszkiewicz, Chemical composition and biological activity of the *Yersinia pestis* envelope substance, *Infect. Immun.* **30:**506–512 (1980).
8. R. C. Williams, H. Gewurz, P. G. Quie, Effects of fraction I from *Yersinia pestis* on phagocytosis in vitro, *J. Infect. Dis.* **126:**235–241 (1972).
9. J. E. Williams, D. N. Harrison, and D. C. Cavanaugh, Cryptic infection of rats with nonencapsulated variants of *Yersinia pestis, Trans. R. Soc. Trop. Med. Hyg.* **69:**171–172 (1975).

10. J. E. Williams, D. N. Harrison, T. J. Quan, J. L. Mullins, A. M. Barnes, and D. C. Cavanaugh, Atypical plague bacilli isolated from rodents, fleas, and man, *Am. J. Public Health* **58:**262–264 (1978).
11. W. A. Janssen and M. J. Surgalla, Plague bacillus: Survival within host phagocytes, *Science* **163:**950–952 (1969).
12. D. C. Cavanaugh and R. Randall, The role of multiplication of *Pasteurella pestis* in mononuclear phagocytes in the pathogenesis of flea-borne plague, *J. Immunol.* **83:**348–363 (1959).
13. T. W. Burrows and G. A. Bacon, The basis of virulence in *Pasteurella pestis:* An antigen determining virulence, *Brit. J. Exp. Pathol.* **37:**481–493 (1956).
14. W. D. Lawton, R. L. Erdman, and M. J. Surgalla, Bisynthesis and purification of V and W antigen in *Pasteurella pestis, J. Immunol.* **91:**179–184 (1963).
15. S. C. Straley and R. R. Brubaker, Localization in *Yersinia pestis* of peptides associated with virulence, *Infect. Immun.* **36:**129–135 (1982).
16. R. J. Zahorchak, W. T. Charnetzky, R. V. Little, and R. R. Brubaker, Consequences of Ca^{2+} deficiency on macromolecular synthesis and adenylate energy charge in *Yersinia pestis, J. Bacteriol.* **139:**792–799 (1979).
17. P. J. Hall and R. R. Brubaker, Pesticin-dependent generation of osmotically stable spheroplast-like structures, *J. Bacteriol.* **136:**786–789 (1978).
18. D. M. Ferber and R. R. Brubaker, Mode of action of pesticin: *N*-acetylglucosaminidase activity, *J. Bacteriol.* **139:**495–501 (1979).
19. R. R. Brubaker, E. D. Beesley, and M. J. Surgalla, *Pasteurella pestis:* Role of pesticin I and iron in experimental plague, *Science* **149:**422–424 (1965).
20. E. D. Beesley, R. R. Brubaker, W. A. Janssen, and M. J. Surgalla, Pesticins III. Expression of coagulase and mechanism of fibrinolysis, *J. Bacteriol.* **94:**19–26 (1967).
20a. A. Wake, H. Morita, and M. Yamamoto, The effect of an iron drug on host response to experimental plague infection, *Jpn. J. Med. Sci. Biol.* **25:**75–84 (1972).
21. C. D. Rail, Roles of metallic ions within an area endemic for the plague bacillus *(Yersinia pestis), Med. Hypothesis* **6:**105–112 (1980).
22. D. A. L. Davies, A specific polysaccharide of *Pasteurella pestis, Biochem. J.* **63:**105–116 (1956).
23. A. B. Foster, D. A. L. Davies, and M. J. Crumpton, Action of periodate on some polysaccharides containing aldoheptose sugars, *Nature* **181:**412–413 (1958).
24. D. C. Ellwood, The 3-deoxy-D-manno-octulosonic acid found in the lipopolysaccharide: *Pasteurella* species, *Biochem. J.* **106:**47p–48p (1968).
25. R. V. Walker, M. G. Barnes, and E. D. Higgins, Composition of and pathophysiology produced by plague endotoxins, *Nature* **209:**1246 (1966).
26. J. L. Hartley, G. A. Adams, and T. G. Tornabene, Chemical and physical properties of lipopolysaccharide of *Yersinia pestis, J. Bacteriol.* **118:**848–854 (1974).
27. E. C. Cocking, J. Keppie, K. Witt, and H. Smith, The chemical basis of the virulence of *Pasteurella pestis* II. The toxicity for guinea pigs and mice of products of *Pasturella pestis, Br. J. Exp. Pathol.* **41:**460–471 (1960).
28. R. V. Walker, Comparative physiopathology of plague endotoxin in mice, guinea pigs, and monkeys, *J. Infect. Dis.* **118:**188–196 (1968).
29. J. M. Albizo and M. J. Surgalla, Isolation and biological characterization of *Pasteurella pestis* endotoxin, *Infect. Immun.* **2:**229–236 (1970).
30. T. Butler and G. Moller, Mitogenic response of mouse spleen cells and gelation of limulus lysate by lipopolysaccharide of *Yersinia pestis* and evidence for neutralization of the lipopolysaccharide by polymyxin B, *Infect. Immun.* **18:**400–404 (1977).

31. R. I. Walker, Detection of an endotoxin-like substance during human plague bacteremia, *Southeast Asian J. Trop. Med. Public Health* **3:**221–224 (1972).
32. T. Butler, J. Levin, D. Q. Cu, and R. I. Walker, Bubonic plague: Detection of endotoxemia with the limulus test, *Ann. Intern. Med.* **79:**642–646 (1973).
33. M. J. Finegold, Pathogenesis of plague: A review of plague deaths in the United States during the last decade, *Am. J. Med.* **45:**549–554 (1968).
34. J. J. Nordlund, R. K. Root, and S. M. Wolff, Studies on the origin of human leukocytic pyrogen, *J. Exp. Med.* **131:**727–743 (1970).
35. H. Prydz and A. C. Allison, Tissue thromboplastin activity of isolated human monocytes, *Thrombosis Haemostasis* **39:**582–584 (1978).
36. R. P. A. Rivers, W. E. Hathaway, and W. L. Weston, The endotoxin-induced coagulant activity of human monocytes, *Br. J. Haematol.* **30:**311–316 (1975).
37. E. Bohn and G. Muller-Berghaus, The effect of leukocyte and platelet transfusion on the activation of intravascular coagulation by endotoxin in granulocytopenic and thrombocytopenic rabbits, *Am J. Pathol.* **84:**239–258 (1976).
38. L. H. Koplik, Experimental production of hemorrhage and vascular lesions in lymph nodes: An extension of the Shwartzman phenomenon, *J. Exp. Med.* **65:**287–302 (1937).
39. S. Kadis, T. C. Montie, and S. J. Ajl, The murine toxin of *Pasteurella pestis:* A study in development, *Bacteriol. Rev.* **30:**177–191 (1960).
40. T. C. Montie and D. B. Montie, Protein toxins of *Pasteurella pestis:* Subunit composition and acid binding, *Biochemistry* **70:**2094–2100 (1971).
41. T. C. Montie and D. B. Montie, Selective detoxification of murine toxin from *Yersinia pestis:* Reaction of heavy metals with essential sulfhydryl and tryptophan residues, *Biochemistry* **12:**4958–4965 (1973).
42. J. H. Rust, D. C. Cavanaugh, S. Kadis, and S. Ajl, Plague toxin: Its effect in vitro and in vivo, *Science* **142:**408–409 (1963).
43. G. J. Hildebrand, J. Ng, E. K. von Metz, and D. M. Eisler, Studies on the mechanism of circulatory failure induced in rats by *Pasteurella pestis* murine toxin, *J. Infect. Dis.* **116:**615–629 (1966).
44. S. D. Brown and T. C. Montie, Beta-adrenergic blocking activity of *Yersinia pestis* murine toxin, *Infect. Immun.* **18:**85–93 (1977).
45. C. E. Davis and K. Arnold, Role of meningococcal endotoxin in meningococcal purpura, *J. Exp. Med.* **140:**159–171 (1974).
46. D. M. Ferber and R. R. Brubaker, Plasmids in *Yersinia pestis, Infect. Immun.* **31:**839–841 (1981).
47. M. J. Finegold, J. J. Petery, R. F. Berendt, and H. R. Adams, Studies on the pathogenesis of plague, *Am. J. Pathol.* **53:**99–111 (1968).
48. M. J. Finegold, Pneumonic plague in monkeys: An electron microscopic study, *Am. J. Pathol.* **54:**167–178 (1969).
48a. T. Butler, Y. S. Fu, L. Furman, C. Almeida, and A. Almeida, Experimental *Yersinia pestis* infeciton in rodents after intragastric inoculation and ingestion of bacteria, *Infect. Immun.* **36:**1160–1167 (1982).
48b. P. B. Carter, L. Lafleur, and S. Toma (eds.), Proceedings of the Third International Symposium on *Yersinia* Infections, *Contrib. Microbiol. Immunol.* **5** (1979).
49. H. H. Mollaret and J. C. Guillon, Contribution à l'étude d'un nouveau groupe de germes *(Yersinia enterocolitica)* proches du bacille de Malassez et Vignal II. Pouvoir pathogène experimental, *Ann. Inst. Pasteur Paris* **109:**608–513 (1965).
50. B. Nilehn, The relationship of incubation temperature to serum bactericidal effect, pathogenicity, and in vivo survival of *Yersinia enterocolitica, Contrib. Microbiol. Immunol.* **2:**85–92 (1973).

51. T. J. Quan, J. L. Meek, K. R. Tsuchiya, B. W. Hudson, and A. M. Barnes, Experimental pathogenicity of recent North American *Yersinia enterocolitica* isolates, *J. Infect. Dis.* **129:**341–344 (1974).
52. P. B. Carter, Pathogenicity of *Yersinia enterocolitica* for mice, *Infect. Immun.* **11:**164–170 (1975).
53. P. B. Carter and F. M. Collins, Experimental *Yersinia enterocolitica* infection in mice: Kinetics of growth, *Infect. Immun.* **9:**851–857 (1974).
54. P. B. Carter, C. F. Varga, and E. E. Keet, New strain of *Yersinia enterocolitica* pathogenic for rodents, *Appl. Microbiol.* **26:**1016–1018 (1973).
55. I. D. Ricciardi, A. D. Pearson, W. G. Suckling, and C. Klein, Long-term fecal excretion and resistance induced in mice infected with *Yersinia enterocolitica, Infect. Immun.* **21:**342–344 (1978).
56. D. A. Schiemann and J. A. Devenish, Virulence of *Yersinia enterocolitica* determined by lethality in Mongolian gerbils and by the Sereny test, *Infect. Immun.* **29:**500–506 (1980).
57. H. Bazin, B. Platteau, M. Janssens, and G. Wauters, Pathogenesis of post-irradiation infections I. *Yersinia enterocolitica* administered to normal and irradiated rats, *Int. J. Radiat. Biol.* **40**(3)**:**277–282 (1981).
58. R. M. Robins-Browne, A. R. Rabson, and H. J. Koornhof, Generalized infection with *Yersinia enterocolitica* and the role of iron, *Contrib. Microbiol. Immunol.* **5:**277–282 (1979).
59. R. E. Smith, A. M. Carey, J. M. Demare, F. M. Hetrick, R. W. Johnston, and W. H. Lee, Evaluation of iron dextran and mucin for enhancement of the virulence of *Yersinia enterocolitica* serotype O:3 in mice, *Infect. Immun.* **34:**550–560 (1981).
60. T. Une, Studies on the pathogenicity of *Yersinia enterocolitica* I. Experimental infection in rabbits, *Microbiol. Immunol.* **7:**349–363 (1977).
61. C. H. Pai, V. Mors, and T. A. Seemayer, Experimental *Yersinia enterocolitica* enteritis in rabbits, *Infect. Immun.* **28:**238–244 (1980).
62. M. Mäki, P. Gronroos, and T. Vesikari, In vitro invasiveness of *Yersinia enterocolitica* isolated from children with diarrhoea, *J. Infect. Dis.* **138:**677–680 (1978).
63. T. Une, Studies on the pathogenicity of *Yersinia enterocolitica* II. Interaction with cultured cells in vitro, *Microbiol. Immunol.* **7:**365–377 (1977).
64. V. Mors and C. H. Pai, Pathogenic properties of *Yersinia enterocolitica, Infect. Immun.* **28:**292–294 (1980).
65. P. Gemski, J. R. Lazere, and T. Casey, Plasmid associated with pathogenicity and calcium dependency of *Yersinia enterocolitica, Infect. Immun.* **27:**682–685 (1980).
66. D. L. Zink, J. C. Feeley, J. G. Wells, C. Vanderzant, J. C. Vickery, W. D. Roof, and G. A. O'Donovan, Plasmid-mediated tissue invasiveness in *Yersinia enterocolitica, Nature* **283:**224–226 (1980).
66a. J. Heesemann, C. Keller, R. Morawa, N. Schmidt, H. J. Siemens, and R. Laufs, Plasmids of human strains of *Yersinia enterocolitica:* Molecular relatedness and possible importance for pathogenesis, *J. Infect. Dis.* **147:**107–115 (1983).
67. B. A. Kay, K. Wachsmuth, and P. Gemski, New virulence-associated plasmid in *Yersinia enterocolitica, J. Clin. Microbiol.* **15:**1161–1163 (1982).
68. C. H. Pai and V. Mors, Production of enterotoxin by *Yersinia enterocolitica, Infect. Immun.* **19:**908–911 (1978).
69. R. M. Robins-Browne, C. S. Still, M. D. Miliotis, and H. J. Koornhof, Mechanism of action of *Yersinia enterocolitica* enterotoxin, *Infect. Immun.* **25:**680–684 (1979).
70. J. M. Boyce, D. J. Evans, D. G. Evans, and H. L. DuPont, Production of heat-stable, methanol-soluble enterotoxin by *Yersinia enterocolitica, Infect. Immun.* **25:**532–537 (1979).

71. M. C. Rao, S. Guandalini, W. J. Laird, and M. Field, Effects of heat-stable enterotoxin of *Yersinia enterocolitica* on ion transport and cyclic guanosine 3′,5′-monophosphate metabolism in rabbit ileum, *Infect. Immun.* **26:**875–878 (1979).
72. K. Okamoto, T. Inoue, H. Ichikawa, Y. Kawamoto, and A. Miyama, Partial purification and characterization of heat-stable enterotoxin produced by *Yersinia enterocolitica, Infect. Immun.* **31:**554–559 (1981).
73. G. Kapperud and G. Langeland, Enterotoxin production at refrigeration temperature by *Yersinia enterocolitica* and *Yersinia enterocolitica*-like bacteria, *Curr. Microbiol.* **5:**119–122 (1981).
74. J. F. Alderete and D. C. Robertson, Purification and chemical characterization of the heat-stable enterotoxin produced by porcine strains of enterotoxigenic *Escherichia coli, Infect. Immun.* **19:**1021–1030 (1978).
75. R. Lallier, S. Lariviere, and S. St-Pierre, *Escherichia coli* heat-stable enterotoxin: Rapid method of purification and some characteristics of the toxin, *Infect. Immun.* **28:**469–474 (1980).
76. B. J. Stoll, R. I. Glass, M. I. Huq, M. U. Khan, H. Banu, and J. Holt, Epidemiologic and clinical features of patients infected with *Shigella* who attended a diarrheal disease hospital in Bangladesh, *J. Infect. Dis.* **146:**177–183 (1982).
77. N. Khuri-Bulos, Enteric fevers in children: The importance of age in the varying clinical picture, *Clin. Pediatr.* **20**(7)**:**448–452 (1981).
78. G. Acker and V. Brade, Activation of human complement by *Yersinia enterocolitica:* Ultrastructural alterations and C3b-deposition, *Zentralbl. Bakteriol. Parasitenkd. Infektionskr. Hyg. Abt. Orig.* **A248:**210–228 (1980).
79. C. H. Pai and L. De Stephano, Serum resistance associated with virulence in *Yersinia enterocolitica, Infect. Immun.* **35:**605–611 (1982).
80. V. Brade and G. Kreuzpaintner, Interaction of lipopolysaccharides and of Lipid A from *Yersinia enterocolitica* with purified guinea pig C3, *Immunobiology* **156:**441–453 (1979).
81. J. Hoffman, B. Lindberg, and R. R. Brubaker, Structural studies of the O-specific side-chains of the lipopolysaccharide from *Yersinia enterocolitica* YE 128, *Carbohydr. Res.* **78:**212–214 (1980).
82. B. Nilehn, Electron microscopic studies on flagellation in different strains of *Yersinia enterocolitica, Acta Pathol. Microbiol. Scand.* **77:**527–541 (1969).
83. I. Kochan, J. T. Kvach, and T. I. Wiles, Virulence-associated acquisition of iron in mammalian serum by *Escherichia coli, J. Infect. Dis.* **135:**623–632 (1977).
84. R. J. Yancey, S. A. L. Breeding, and C. E. Lankford, Enterochelin (enterobactin): Virulence factor for *Salmonella typhimurium, Infect. Immun.* **24:**174–180 (1979).
85. K. Melby, S. Slordahl, T. J. Gutteberg, and S. A. Nordbo, Septicemia due to *Yersinia enterocolitica* after oval overdoses of iron, *Br. Med. J.* **285:**467–468 (1982).
86. M. Leirisalo, H. Repo, A. Tilikainen, T. U. Kosunnen, and O. Laitinen, Chemotaxis in *Yersinia* arthritis: HLA-B27 positive neutrophils show high stimulated motility in vitro, *Arthritis Rheum.* **24:**1036–1044 (1980).
87. T. Une, Studies on the pathogenicity of *Yersinia enterocolitica* III. Comparative studies between *Y. enterocolitica* and *Y. pseudotuberculosis, Microbiol. Immunol.* **21:**505–516 (1977).
88. A. Bovallius and G. Nilsson, Ingestion and survial of *Y. pseudotuberculosis* in HeLa cells, *Can. J. Microbiol.* **21:**1997–2007 (1975).
89. K. Samuelsson, B. Lindberg, and R. R. Brubaker, Structure of O-specific side chains of lipopolysaccharide of *Yersinia pseudotuberculosis, J. Bacteriol.* **117:**1010–1016 (1974).

90. R. P. Gorshkova, N. A. Komandrova, A. I. Kalinovsky, and Y. S. Ovodov, Structural studies on the O-specific polysaccharide side-chains of *Yersinia pseudotuberculosis,* Type III, lipopolysaccharides, *Eur. J. Biochem.* **107:**131–135 (1980).
91. R. R. Brubaker, Growth of *Pasteurella pseudotuberculosis* in simulated intracellular and extracellular environments, *J. Infect. Dis.* **117:**403–417 (1967).

6

Diagnosis and Treatment

In this section, I shall present and discuss recent work that relates to selected aspects of the diagnosis and treatment of *Yersinia* infections. Plague will be considered separately from the other yersiniae because the isolation and identification of *Yersinia pestis* is a more simple laboratory exercise owing to its presence in normally sterile body fluids. Selective media and cold enrichment are often necessary, on the other hand, to recover the other yersiniae from the multiplicity of microbes present in the normal stool. The treatment of plague is similarly more straightforward because antibiotics are lifesaving in plague, whereas the efficacy of antibiotic treatment in the other yersinioses is less well established.

6.1. THE DIAGNOSIS OF PLAGUE

6.1.1. Clinical Diagnosis

The essential first step in the diagnosis of plague is to suspect the diagnosis in any person with fever who lives in a known endemic area of the world or who has visited a known endemic area within the past few days. The diagnosis should be more strongly suspected if the patient with fever also has a painful bubo, cough, or signs of meningitis. Once the diagnosis is suspected, a physician should proceed to establish the diagnosis by bacteriological methods.

6.1.2. Bacteriological Diagnosis

A bacteriological diagnosis is made readily in most patients by smear and culture of a bubo aspirate. The aspirate is obtained by inserting a 20-gauge needle on a 10 cc syringe containing 1 cc of sterile saline solution into the bubo and withdrawing several times until the saline becomes blood tinged. Because the bubo does not contain liquid pus, it may be necessary to inject some of the saline and immediately reaspirate it. Drops of the aspirate should be placed onto microscope slides and air-dried for both gram and Wayson's stains. The gram stain will reveal polymorphonuclear leukocytes and gram-negative coccobacilli and bacilli ranging from 1 to 2 μm in length. Wayson's stain is prepared by mixing 0.2 g of basic fuchsin (90% dye content) with 0.75 g of methylene blue (90% dye content) in 20 ml of 95% ethyl alcohol. This preparation is then poured slowly into 200 ml of 5% phenol. A smear, after being fixed for 2 min in absolute methanol, is stained for 10 to 20 sec in Wayson's stain, washed with water, and dried. *Y. pestis* organisms appear as light blue bacilli with dark blue polar bodies, and the remainder of the slide has a contrasting pink counterstain.[1]

The aspirate, blood, and other appropriate fluids should be inoculated onto blood and MacConkey agar plates and into infusion broth. Like all other Enterobacteriaceae, *Y. pestis* is oxidase-negative, reduces nitrate, and ferments glucose. The organism is identified in triple-sugar–iron agar by an alkaline slant and acid butt without gas or H_2S, by negative reactions for Christensen's urea and indole, by failure to utilize citrate, and by nonmotility at both 25°C and 37°C.[2] The ability of *Y. pestis* to ferment carbohydrates, when compared to the other yersiniae, is more limited, being restricted to only glucose and trehalose. *Y. pestis* grows more slowly than other Enterobacteriaceae on agar plates, forming pinpoint colonies after 24 hr at 35°C. This organism grows at an optimal rate at 28°C.

A more rapid bacteriological diagnosis of plague can be made by applying a fluorescent antibody test directly to smears of the bubo aspirate, sputum, or spinal fluid. Specific antisera with antibodies against Fraction I of *Y. pestis* have been prepared and conjugated with fluorocein isothiocyanate. Thus, an immediate diagnosis is possible. This technique is available now at the Plague Branch of the Centers for Disease Control in Fort Collins, Colorado, U.S.

Several other diagnostic aids for the identification of *Y. pestis,* which are not in general use, have been developed and can be applied in special situations. One of these is the use of specific bacteriophages which lyse *Y. pestis* organisms on a bacteriological agar plate.[3] Bacteriophage lysis can be used to confirm the identification of *Y. pestis,* but is not necessary in a laboratory that has differential biochemical tests available. The phages obtained from *Y. pestis* are not absolutely specific for *Y. pestis* and do produce lysis of certain other Enterobacteriaceae. Nunes and Suassuna[3] showed great specificity can be achieved by diluting the phage particles and differentiating among patterns of partial lysis.

Other variations in bacteriological media can enable one to distinguish virulent *Y. pestis* from avirulent strains. Surgalla *et al.*[4] summarized information about these media. Antiserum with antibodies against Fraction I have been incorporated into agar media. After the growth of bacterial colonies and exposure of the agar to chloroform vapor, precipitation rings are visible around colonies of *Y. pestis* with Fraction I antigen. Organisms that produce pesticin can be detected by overlaying agar on which bacteria have been grown and arrested with chloroform vapor with another agar layer containing type I *Yersinia pseudotuberculosis*. Clear zones of inhibition of *Y. pseudotuberculosis* around colonies of *Y. pestis* indicate the presence of pesticin production. The V and W antigens can be detected in *Y. pestis* by showing inhibition of growth on magnesium oxalate agar at 37°C. Virulent strains produce a pigment which can be detected by growing bacteria on an agar containing galactose and Congo-red stain. Pigmented strains produce red colonies on this agar. Finally, the fibrinolytic factor of virulent *Y. pestis* can be detected by culturing bacteria on a film of opalescent fibrin and looking for clear zones around the colonies.

Quan *et al.*[5] described a test to detect isocitrate lyase activity in bacterial colonies. This test can be performed in only 20 min to give a presumptive diagnosis of *Y. pestis* before other definite biochemical tests are completed. They found that 1695 strains gave positive results, but no other Enterobacteriaceae tested were positive.

Electron microscopy has been applied to cultures of *Y. pestis* to demonstrate the ultrastructure of virulent organisms.[6] When grown at 37°C for 72 hr, scanning electron microscopy showed a shaggy surface with particles that represent Fraction I antigen, whereas the same strain grown at 22°C showed a smooth surface.

In addition to the classical virulent strains, atypical strains lacking one or more of the virulence factors have been isolated in nature.[7] Because these strains are less pathogenic in laboratory animals than the fully virulent strains, the isolation of these variants from patients has less certain diagnostic significance. One example is a strain of *Y. pestis* isolated from the bubo of a 29-year-old Vietnamese woman in 1974. This strain was nonpigmented, but had produced a fever of 39°C, the bubo, and an illness that lasted 2 days (T. Butler, unpublished observations). Other strains isolated from rats in Java were negative for the V and W antigens.[7] It has been speculated that these less virulent variants of *Y. pestis* may be responsible for mild cases of plague in populations of rodents or man and also for producing immunity in humans after causing asymptomatic infections.

6.1.3. Electrophoresis of *Yersinia pestis*

There exists no serotyping scheme or phage-typing scheme to separate strains of *Y. pestis* into different genetic groups that might permit epidemiological tracing of sources of individual infections or outbreaks of infection. Hudson, Quan, and colleagues used electrophoresis to define variant types.[8,9] They used discontinuous acrylamide gel electrophoresis and photometric techniques to obtain profiles of each strain. They identified 18 to 25 visible protein bands from aqueous extracts of acetone powders of each strain. Analysis of 161 isolates from Asia, southeast Asia, Indonesia, Africa, North America, and South America resulted in the identification of 11 major electropherotype groups that represented major protein variants. The geographic distribution of the 11 electropherotype groups corresponded to known routes of dispersion of *Y. pestis* during the present pandemic,[10] suggesting that this method of genetic typing may have value as an epidemiological tool in the future.

6.1.4. Serological Techniques

6.1.4.1. Passive Hemagglutination (PHA) to Detect Antibodies against Fraction IA Antigen of *Yersinia pestis*

This is the most widely used and accepted serological test for plague in the world today. It has been standardized by the World Health Organization (WHO) and is recommended for diagnostic confirmation of human cases, for seroepidemiology, and for the detection of enzootic plague in animal populations.[11]

The technique of extraction of Fraction IA antigen has been described by Baker *et al.*[12] and the method of sensitizing sheep red blood cells by the WHO Expert Committee on Plague.[13] Briefly, cultures of *Y. pestis* are dried with acetone washes. A water-soluble extract is made by suspending the bacilli in 2.5% NaCl solution saturated with toluene and allowing this suspension to stand at room temperature for 24 hr. The bacteria are removed by centrifugation and the supernatant is dialyzed. Agar protein is removed by adding saturated ammonium sulfate to give a concentration of 0.25 saturation. After discarding the precipitate, saturated ammonium sulfate is added to the supernatant to give a concentration of 0.3 saturation. The precipitate is collected by centrifugation and this is Fraction IA antigen. It is further purified by dissolving in water and precipitating proteins again with ammonium sulfate at a concentration of 0.25 saturation and then reprecipitating Fraction IA antigen with ammonium sulfate at a concentration of 0.3 saturation. This precipitate is dissolved in water, dialyzed against water, and dried. Sheep red blood cells are collected in Alsever's solution, washed, and fixed in glutaraldehyde. The cells are exposed to tannic acid and sensitized with Fraction IA antigen of *Y. pestis* in a final concentration of 100 μg antigen/ml. The PHA test is performed by microtiter technique and controlled by concomitant passive hemagglutination inhibition testing (PHI). Into each well of the PHA microtiter plate is pipetted 0.025 ml of normal rabbit serum (NRS) 1 : 100 in 0.9% NaCl solution, and into each well of the PHI control is placed 0.025 ml of NRS 1 : 100 in 0.9% NaCl solution containing 100 μg antigen/ml. Using a microdiluter with a volume of 0.025 ml, test sera and control sera are delivered to both PHA and PHI wells and 11 two-fold dilutions are made of each serum in a row. Finally, 0.025 ml of sensitized red blood cells 0.5% by volume in NRS 1 : 250 in 0.9% NaCl solution are delivered to all wells. The plates are swirled, covered, and allowed to stand overnight at 4°C. The highest dilutions of sera that show hemagglutination are recorded and compared to the PHI titers. Sera with PHA titers of $\geqslant$ 1 : 16 are readsorbed with sheep red blood cells and retested. Sera are considered positive only when repeated testing shows a PHA titer of $\geqslant$ 1 : 16 that is about eight-fold or more above the PHI titer.

A modification of the PHA, which was suggested by Suzuki *et al.*,[14] employed 2-mercaptoethanol treatment of sera to inactive antibodies of the IgM class. This method has the advantage of distinguishing between antibodies that form early during infection (primarily IgM) and those that persist later into convalescence (primarily IgG).

6.1.4.2. Latex Agglutination

Suzuki and co-workers[15] reported that Fraction I antigen could be coated to polystyrene latex particles. Using either a slide or microtiter technique, they showed that this test had both sensitivity and specificity that were comparable to that of the PHA test. This latex agglutination test has the possible advantages over the PHA method that the latex agglutination antigen was stable for at least 12 months and that latex particles are easier to obtain and prepare than are sheep red blood cells.

6.1.4.3. Other Serological Tests

Cavanaugh *et al.*[16] reported an application of the newer enzyme-linked immunoabsorbent assay (ELISA) to plague serology. Briefly, Fraction I antigen of *Y. pestis* was allowed to adhere to the plastic wells of an ELISA plate. Test sera in serial dilutions are added and allowed to incubate for 30 min at 37°C. Unabsorbed serum antibodies are washed out and horseradish peroxidase that is conjugated to species-specific antiimmunoglobulin is added to the wells. After washing again, the substrate solution containing 5-aminosalicylic acid is added. Enzymatic activity is measured by reading the optical density of each plate well at 455 nm. This ELISA technique gave a simple and reproducible method for detecting plague antibodies in sera of humans and rats. Its advantage over the PHA test is that both IgG and IgM antibodies can be separately measured by the use of class-specific antiimmunoglobulins, which are commercially available.

Another newer serological test for plague is the solid phase radioimmunoassay (SPRIA) that has been described by Hudson and co-workers.[17] Like the ELISA test, it gave results that were comparable to the PHA and could also distinguish between IgM and IgG antibody classes.

6.2. DIAGNOSIS OF *YERSINIA ENTEROCOLITICA* and *YERSINIA PSEUDOTUBERCULOSIS* INFECTIONS

6.2.1. Clinical Diagnosis

The diagnosis of yersiniosis should be suspected in every person with fever and abdominal pain. The suspicion of the diagnosis should be especially strong in persons with these syndromes who live in the known endemic areas of Canada, New York, Belgium, France, Sweden, Norway, and Finland.

During epidemics of appendicitislike diseases or diarrhea, yersiniosis should be always considered. Furthermore, the diagnosis should be entertained in patients with sepsis in the setting of prior liver disease and in patients with the immunological reactions of arthritis and erythema nodosum. A recently published book by E. J. Bottone has detailed information on the clinical and laboratory diagnosis of *Y. enterocolitica*.[18]

6.2.2. Bacteriological Diagnosis

The isolation and identification of yersiniae in the laboratory from normally sterile tissues is straightforward according to standard bacteriological principles.[2] Isolation from stool requires selective media and sometimes cold enrichment, which will be described below. Like other Enterobacteriaceae, the yersiniae grow on bile-salt-containing agars such as MacConkey agar, ferment glucose, are oxidase-negative, and reduce nitrates. On MacConkey agar, these bacteria produce colorless lactose-nonfermenting colonies. The typical strains of yersiniae give positive reactions in Christensen's urea and negative reactions for citrate utilization. On the triple-sugar–iron agar, *Y. enterocolitica* produces an acid slant and acid butt without gas or H_2S, whereas *Y. pseudotuberculosis* produces an alkaline slant and acid butt without gas or H_2S. This difference is due to the fact that *Y. enterocolitica* ferments sucrose. These biochemical tests will allow presumptive identification of these two species. Further testing is advisable to confirm the identification, and some of the helpful tests that allow a laboratory to distinguish among the three species of yersiniae are shown in Table 6.1. The tests that distinguish *Y.*

TABLE 6.1
Distinguishing Features of Members of the Genus *Yersinia*

Test	*Y. pestis*	*Y. enterocolitica*	*Y. pseudotuberculosis*
Motility			
25°C	−	+	+
37°C	−	−	−
Christensen's urea	−	+	+
Ornithine decarboxylase	−	+	−
Acid produced from:			
Sucrose	−	+	−
Rhamnose	−	−	+
Melibiose	−	−	+
Cellobiose	−	+	−

TABLE 6.2
Biotypes of *Yersinia enterocolitica* According to Wauter's Scheme

Test	Biotypes 1	2	3	4	5
Lecithinase	+	−	−	−	−
Indole production	+	+	−	−	−
Xylose fermentation at 25°C	+	+	+	−	−
Lactose fermentation at 25°C	+	+	+	−	−
Nitrate reduction	+	+	+	+	−
Trehalose fermentation	+	+	+	+	−
Ornithine decarboxylase at 25°C	+	+	+	+	−
Beta-galactosidase	+	+	+	+	−

enterocolitica from *Y. pseudotuberculosis* are ornithine decarboxylase and acid fermentation of sucrose, rhamnose, melibiose, and cellobiose.

Thus, the typical strains of *Y. enterocolitica* are positive for sucrose and cellobiose and negative for rhamnose, and melibiose. Additional biochemical tests were originally used by Wauters[(18a)] in 1970 to separate *Y. enterocolitica* into five biotypes. This schema for biotyping is shown in Table 6.2. Most of the human isolates from Europe belong to Biotype 4, but isolates of other biotypes have been found in the environment and occasionally in humans. A modification of this scheme for biotyping has been employed in Europe by Bercovier *et al.*[(19)] and it adds a sixth biotype to the list, designated 1B.

In addition to the typical *Y. enterocolitica* strains that are sucrose-positive and rhamnose-negative, variant strains have been isolated from both human and environmental sources. These organisms are still in the process of being definitively classified, and the scheme in Table 6.3 has been proposed. Brenner

TABLE 6.3
Groups of *Yersinia enterocolitica* and *Yersinia enterocolitica*-like Organisms Showing DNA Relatedness[a]

	Y. enterocolitica	*Y. intermedia*	*Y. frederiksenii*	*Y. kristensenii* or *Y. ruckeri*
Sucrose	+	+	+	−
Rhamnose	−	+	+	−
Raffinose	−	+	−	−
Melibiose	−	+	−	−
α-Methylglucoside	−	+	−	−

[a] + Indicates fermentation of carbohydrate.

and co-workers[20,21] have carried out extensive studies of DNA relatedness by hybridizing DNA of different strains at different temperatures. They consider strains with 70% or more relatedness to belong to the same species and strains that are 35% or more related to belong to the same genus. They found that strains of *Y. pestis* and *Y. pseudotuberculosis* were more than 80% related, indicating that these species are genetically so similar that they could be considered as the same species. Accordingly, they found that strains of *Yersinia intermedia* and *Yersinia frederiksenii* were about 60% related to typical *Y. enterocolitica,* and thus they should be in the same genus but not the same species. Strains of *Yersinia ruckeri* were only 30% related to *Y. enterocolitica,* indicating perhaps a more tenuous right to belong to the same genus. However, the guanosine and cytosine content of these strains were very close to other yersiniae.

The pathogenicity of these strains has been questioned. Bottone *et al.*[22] reported isolating 12 strains of *Y. intermedia* from human sources, which were not the usual mesenteric lymphadenitis cases. Four of these isolations were from the eye, three from stool, two from urine, and one each from a wound and the trachea. Chester *et al.*[23] reported the isolation of 13 atypical strains, which fit the currently used criteria of *Y. intermedia*. They came from human and environmental sources and were serotyped as O:16, O:17, and untypable. *Y. ruckeri* has been implicated as the cause of red-mouth disease in salmon and trout. Other workers, including Baker and Farmer,[24] use the species name *Y. kristensenii* in place of *Y. ruckeri*.

Bottone *et al.*[25] have tested many strains of *Y. enterocolitica* for bacteriocin production and found that only *Y. intermedia* strains produced bacteriocin. The bacteriocin was active against only certain strains of *Y. enterocolitica* and *Y. frederiksenii,* and was produced only at 25°C. The specificity of the bacteriocin for members of the genus *Yersinia* was used as an additional argument for the placement of *Y. intermedia* into the same genus.

Other atypical features of *Y. enterocolitica* have been attributed to plasmids. Cornelis *et al.*[26] isolated a strain from the throat of a patient. This strain fermented both lactose and raffinose, properties that were conferred by a 33-megadalton plasmid. Another atypical feature reported in *Y. enterocolitica* is hemolysis of blood agar in the presence of lecithin. This was noted by Tsubokura *et al.*[27] in a Biotype 1 strain and was subsequently found in 85 of 202 strains, which included typical strains also. The hemolytic activity was attributed to the enzymatic action of phospholipase A and lipase on lecithin.

In addition to serotyping and biotyping, methods of phage typing have been used to separate strains of *Y. enterocolitica* further. A complex scheme was used by Baker *et al.*[24] that employed a composite set of 24 phages. These phages were obtained from pooled raw sewage in North Carolina and Georgia and were lytic for yersiniae. The phage types agreed well with serotyping and epidemiological results in studies of defined outbreaks of *Y. enterocolitica* illness. In Spain, Calvo *et al.*[28] collected from water seven phages that were active on *Y. enterocolitica*. These waterborne phages and phages from lysogenic strains were lytic only to *Y. enterocolitica* strains grown at 25°C.

The feces of patients with diarrhea or abdominal pain should be cultured. According to Highsmith *et al.*[29] Salmonella Shigella (SS) agar was found to be unreliable for supporting growth of all strains. For direct isolation, the stool specimen or rectal swab should be plated onto MacConkey agar and incubated at 25°C for 48 hr. Lactose-negative colonies should be screened on triple-sugar–iron agar, in Christensen's urea, and for motility at both 25°C and 36°C. Suspected isolates can be confirmed by further biochemical tests.[30,31]

This method of direct isolation of *Y. enterocolitica* is effective when there are large numbers of organisms in the stool in relation to other organisms such as *Escherichia coli,* which may overgrow the yersiniae on MacConkey agar plates. This method detects well the recognized human pathogenic serotypes O:3, O:8, and O:9. Other strains, however, such as strains belonging to Biotype 1, atypical strains, and other strains that are present in lesser numbers, will not be detected unless cold enrichment is used. Cold enrichment takes advantage of the fact that *Y. enterocolitica* will survive and even multiply slowly under aerobic conditions at 4°C, whereas most other fecal bacteria die off or are held stationary. Cold enrichment is especially useful to detect smaller numbers of organisms that may be present in convalescent or asymptomatic cases.[32] Highsmith *et al.*[29] suggest placing a rectal swab into 5 ml of 0.067 M phosphate buffer at pH 7.6. After 21 days of refrigeration at 4°C, O.1 ml of the buffer is subcultured onto MacConkey agar. Weissfeld and Sonnenwirth[33] suggest a similar method of inoculating stool into phosphate-buffered saline at pH 8.6. This is kept at 4°C for 3 weeks and is subcultured weekly onto MacConkey agar and cellobiose–arginine–lysine agar (CAL). The plates are held for 48 hr at room temperature and examined for typical colonies.[34] On CAL agar the colonies of *Y. enterocolitica* are pink to red and easily recognized. Using a slightly different method of cold enrichment, Eiss[35] placed specimens into nutrient broth. After 2 and 5 days of incubation at 4°C, he plated the broth onto MacConkey agar for 2 days at 25°C. He was able by this method to increase the yield of isolation of *Y. enterocolitica* serotypes O:3, O:8, and O:9 by about 40%.

Using a different cold enrichment medium of 10 ml of phosphate-buffered saline containing 1% mannitol at pH 7.3, Weissfeld and Sonnenwirth,[36] recovered *Y. enterocolitica* from five patients. All had abdominal pain and three had diarrhea. The strains were all Biotype 1 and belonged to serotypes O:5, O:6,30, and O:7,8. None of the five were isolated directly without cold enrichment; one was isolated after 7 days of enrichment and the others after 14 days. From another patient in the United States, *Y. enterocolitica* serotype O:6 was isolated by cold enrichment.[37]

Alternative methods to the cumbersome cold enrichment have been tested by Weissfeld and Sonnenwirth.[38] They treated fecal specimens with 0.5% potassium hydroxide (KOH) to eliminate *E. coli,* klebsiellae, and *Pseudomonas*. This was compared with freezing stools at −70°C and then transferring to *m*-tetrathionate broth and then to selenite broth before plating for culture. The KOH treatment gave a higher yield of *Y. enterocolitica* recovery than did the freeze shock method. Thus, KOH treatment can be considered as an alternative to cold enrichment.

Certain media have been developed to aid in the rapid detection of *Y. enterocolitica* from stools. Schiemann[39] reported good results with a selective agar called cefsulodin–irgason–novobiocin agar (CIN), showing higher yields from stool than SS and MacConkey agar. Bowen and Kominos[40] used a pectin agar, taking advantage of the fact that only yersiniae and certain klebsiellae are pectinolytic. Colonies characteristically form depressions and sink into the agar. Other techniques have been developed to identify *Y. enterocolitica* in water by membrane filter[41] and from food.[42]

6.2.3. Serological Techniques

Antibodies against yersiniae have been detected by a variety of techniques. The technique most widely used is the tube agglutination assay (Widal). To prepare the antigen for this assay, bacteria are grown, washed, and placed in formalin at a final concentration of 0.5%. Winblad *et al.*[42a] found that the O antigen works more satisfactorily than the OH antigen. The O antigen is prepared by heating washed whole bacteria in saline at 120°C for 2.5 hr, followed by repeated washing and resuspension in saline. Sera are diluted and reacted with antigen in a tube to form an agglutination reaction. A simplified and improved agglutination test was developed by Ricciardi *et al.*[43] who boiled cultures of *Y. enterocolitica* serotype O:5,27 stained with triphenyl-tetrazolium chloride. This single antigen gave good cross-reactions with nine different O serotypes and gave little or no cross-reactivity with *Y. pseudotuberculosis* and *Brucella*. Another technique that has been successfully employed is the indirect hemagglutination test using sheep erythrocytes sensitized with heated bacterial extracts.

Newer methods that have been used to detect anti-*Yersinia* antibodies include the ELISA and solid-phase radioimmunoassays. Granfors[44] used the O antigen of a strain O:9 and the formalinized OH antigen of a strain O:3 and of *Y. pseudotuberculosis* group IA to place into wells of the microplate. Antibodies of IgM, IgG, and IgA classes were detected by class specific rabbit antihuman gammaglobulins. The results correlated well with tube agglutination results. The IgM antibodies disappeared during the first 3 months, whereas the IgG antibodies persisted for at least 5 months. In patients with arthritis, the IgA antibodies persisted from 9 to 14 months. The ELISA was used by Gripenberg *et al.*[45] to detect antibodies against lipopolysaccharide of *Y. enterocolitica* serotype O:3. In a modification of the ELISA, Lange *et al.*[46] used the diffusion-in-gel ELISA to detect antibodies against lipopolysaccharide from *Y. enterocolitica* serotype O:3. Good correlation was found between the direct agglutination method and IgG antibody class only.

Granfors *et al.*[47] have developed a SPRIA to detect antibodies. They used heated or formalinized whole bacteria of *Y. enterocolitica* serotypes O:3 and O:9 and *Y. pseudotuberculosis* group IA as antigens which were coated onto polystyrene balls. Sera were exposed to the balls and antibodies of IgM and IgG classes detected by the capacity of the exposed balls to bind ^{125}I-labeled sheep antibodies to human immunoglobulins. The SPRIA results correlated well with direct agglutination in specificity by the finding that all sera that were negative in agglutination were negative also in the SPRIA. However, the SPRIA was somewhat less sensitive, as shown by the result that 10 of 202 sera with agglutination titers $\geqslant 1:80$ gave negative SPRIA results. The IgG antibodies persisted longer than the IgM antibodies.

6.2.4. Problems with Specificity of *Yersinia* Serology

Three lines of evidence have cast doubt on the specificity of *Yersinia* serology. Common enterobacterial antigen has been found in *Y. enterocolitica*, cross-reactions between *Brucella* species and *Yersinia* have been documented, and patients with a variety of thyroid diseases have been reported to show elevated anti-*Yersinia* antibody titers.

The common enterobacterial antigen (CA) is defined as an ethanol-soluble fraction of supernatants of heated bacterial cultures. Bacteria that belong to the family Enterobacteriaceae possess this antigen. Maeland and Digranes[(48)] reported that *Y. enterocolitica* also possesses the CA. The same investigators showed that 200 sera from blood donors in Norway showed antibodies against *Y. enterocolitica* serotypes O:3 and O:9 by indirect hemagglutination.[(49)] The same sera contained also antibodies against the CA, and CA itself could inhibit the hemagglutination reaction in 23 of 30 tested donor sera. This indicated that the anti-*Yersinia* antibodies detected in most of the normal donors' sera were directed against CA and probably originated from exposure to enterobacteria other than yersiniae. On the other hand, some of the donor sera and sera from five patients were not inhibited by CA and agglutinated heated bacteria of serotype O:3. This work has provided valuable information on the limited specificity of some serological tests and a method for improving specificity.

In 1969, Ahvonen *et al.* showed that serological cross-reaction occurred between *Brucella abortus* and *Y. enterocolitica* O:9.[(50)] The antigenic determinants common to these two bacteria have been shown to be present in the lipopolysaccharides. Work by Hurvell[(51,52)] and Hurvell and Lindberg[(53)] has clarified the nature of this cross-reactivity. Lipopolysaccharides that were extracted from both bacteria elicited antibodies in rabbits that cross-reacted with the lipopolysaccharide of the other bacterium in an agglutination test which used whole bacteria as the antigen. In immunodiffusion studies which used antiserum against whole bacterial cells, they showed that the lipopolysaccharide antigens gave good precipitin lines after the antigen had been treated by lipolytic and proteolytic enzymes. However, periodate treatment of the antigen destroyed the precipitating ability, indicating that the carbohydrate portion of the lipopolysaccharide was essential for precipitation. They found that both bacterial lipopolysaccharides contained glucose and galactose as monosaccharides but that *B. abortus* contained mannose and *Y. enterocolitica* contained heptose. They concluded that the cross-reactivity resided in the O-specific polysaccharides of the bacteria. Using an immunolectrophoretic technique, Hurvell was able to distinguish antibodies raised in rabbits against either *B. abortus* or *Y. enterocolitica*.[(52)] Although the agglutination tests gave results that indicated complete cross-reactivity, the pattern of electrophoretic precipitate showed multiple distinct precipitin lines when *Y. enterocolitica* antigen was reacted with homologous antiserum.

Other organisms that may have cross-reacting antigens with yersiniae are *Rickettsia* species. From Israel, Schlesinger *et al.*[54] reported a patient with fever and terminal ileitis who had a high agglutinin titer against *Y. enterocolitica* serotype O:3 which fell after the illness. At the same time there was a significant IgM titer against spotted fever, suggesting the possibility of cross-reactivity of these antigens.

An unexpected and remarkable discovery was finding the association of anti-*Yersinia* antibodies and thyroid diseases. This was first reported in 1974 in Denmark by Bech *et al.*[55] They reported that in 185 patients, of which 142 had thyrotoxicosis and 43 had nontoxic goiter, the incidence of elevated agglutinating antibodies against *Y. enterocolitica* serotype O:3 was 47–67%. This compared with a 17% incidence of elevated agglutinins in healthy controls. In the United States, Shenkman and Bottone[56] also found this association. In healthy controls, less than 8% had agglutinins against *Y. enterocolitica* serotypes O:3, O:8, and O:9. In 67 patients with a variety of thyroid disorders, 48 (75%) had agglutinin titers of $\geq 1:8$. Most of the patients had Grave's disease, but others with elevated titers also had Hashimoto's thyroiditis, idiopathic primary hypothyroidism, autonomous adenoma, and nontoxic goiter. There was no relation between antithyroid antibody titers and anti-*Yersinia* titers. There was also no relation between the activity of the thyroid disease and the presence of the *Yersinia* agglutinins. None of the patients had signs or symptoms of intestinal infection. Reynolds *et al.*[57] reported another example of this association in a 13-year-old girl with exophthalmos who became hyperthyroid and had an anti-*Yersinia* antibody titer of 1 : 160. She did not have thyroid autoantibodies except for an antithyroglobulin antibody titer of 1 : 40.

This association between *Yersinia* agglutinins and thyroid disease has raised intriguing possibilities. The patients with thyroid disease have not revealed epidemiologic or clinical evidence of prior *Yersinia* infection. Nevertheless, it is possible that they had asymptomatic intestinal infections that generated antibodies which cross-reacted with thyroid tissue. The failure of the studies, however, to show an association between the titers of the *Yersinia* agglutinins and thyroid autoantibodies suggest that the same antibodies do not have both specificities. Both antibodies against *Yersinia* and against thyroid tissue could have arisen separately as a result of a *Yersinia* infection, and one type of antibody is detectable for longer than the other, thus explaining the failure of studies to show correlations in titers. The other interesting explanation for the association of *Yersinia* agglutinins and thyroid disease is that thyroid tissue (normal or damaged) shares some antigen(s) with *Y. enterocolitica*. After thyroid disease occurs and autoantibodies develop, there are also antibodies that cross-react with *Y. enterocolitica* in the absence of a prior infection.

6.3. TREATMENT OF PLAGUE

6.3.1. Antibiotics

Untreated plague has an estimated mortality rate of greater than 50% and can evolve into a fulminant course of septic shock. Therefore, the early institution of effective antibiotic therapy is mandatory immediately after appropriate cultures have been taken. In 1948, streptomycin was shown to be the drug of choice for the treatment of plague by reducing mortality to less than 5%.[58] No other drug has been demonstrated to be better or less toxic. Streptomycin should be administered intramuscularly in two divided doses daily totaling 30 mg/kg per day for 10 days. Most patients show improvement rapidly and become afebrile in about 3 days. The 10-day course of streptomycin is recommended to prevent relapses because viable bacteria have been isolated from buboes of patients during convalescence. The risk of vestibular damage and hearing loss caused by streptomycin is minimal during a 10-day course. It should be used cautiously, however, in pregnancy, in older patients who would have trouble adapting to vestibular damage, and in patients who already have hearing difficulty. In these patients, the course of streptomycin can be reasonably shortened to 3 days after the patient becomes afebrile. Renal injury as a result of streptomycin therapy is rare with the usual clinical dosages, but renal function should be monitored. If the serum creatinine rises significantly, the dose of streptomycin should be reduced. In mild renal failure the recommended dose is 1.5 g per day and in advanced renal failure 0.5 g every 3 days. Most of the preparations of streptomycin available in the United States are in an oil base and can be administered only intramuscularly.

For patients allergic to streptomycin or in whom an oral drug is strongly preferred, tetracycline is a satisfactory alternative to streptomycin.[59] Tetracycline is administered orally in a dose of 2 to 4 g per day in four divided doses for 10 days. Tetracycline is contraindicated in children younger than 7 years and in pregnant women in order to avoid staining of developing teeth. It is also contraindicated in renal failure.

For patients with meningitis, who will require a drug that penetrates well into the cerebrospinal fluid, and for patients with profound hypotension, in whom an intramuscular injection may not be well absorbed, chloramphenicol should be administered intravenously with a loading dose of 25 mg/kg followed by 60 mg/kg per day in four divided doses. After clinical improvement, chloramphenicol should be continued orally to complete a total course of 10 days. The dosage may be reduced to 30 mg/kg per day to reduce the magnitude of bone marrow suppression, which is reversible after completion of therapy. The irreversible bone marrow aplasia associated with chloramphenicol is so rare (incidence is estimated as 1 in 40,000 patients) that its consideration should not deter the use of chloramphenicol for patients seriously ill with plague infection.

Other antimicrobial drugs have been used in plague with varying success. These include sulfonamides, trimethoprim–sulfamethoxazole,[(60)] kanamycin, and ampicillin. These drugs, however, all appear to be either less effective or more toxic than streptomycin and should, therefore, not be chosen for the treatment of plague.

Antibiotic resistance in human isolates of *Y. pestis* has never been reported nor has resistance emerged during antibiotic therapy. The three antibiotics streptomycin, tetracycline, and chloramphenicol given alone are clinically very effective, and relapses are exceedingly rare. Therefore, there is no rationale for using multiple antibiotics to treat plague.

Use of Ampicillin in Experimental Plague Infection

Experimental studies were carried out (T. Butler and M. R. Jacobs, unpublished observations) to test whether ampicillin was an effective antibiotic. Streptomycin is not an ideal antibiotic because of its potential nephrotoxicity and vestibular toxicity. Ampicillin has been given to several patients with plague before the correct diagnosis was made, and one of these patients with plague meningitis improved during 4 days of treatment.[(60)]

Three strains of *Y. pestis* were used: Strain 5 isolated from the blood of a patient in Brazil in 1977 and strains 14 and 18 isolated from buboes of patients in Vietnam in 1974. Bacteria were cultured in 0.5% NaCl in peptone broth for 5 hr at 37°C and diluted according to a McFarland turbidity standard for inoculation. The actual inoculum size was verified by viable colony counts on nutrient agar on the next day. All these strains killed most mice within 8 days after subcutaneous injection of 10^3 bacteria, producing typical disease with heavily infected blood, spleen, and liver.

Susceptibility of *Y. pestis* was tested by both the method of agar diffusion and tube dilution in broth. Susceptibility to ampicillin was tested in heart infusion broth and to streptomycin in nutrient broth. Tubes that contained 1 ml of broth were inoculated with 10^5 bacteria and were read for turbidity after 24 and 48 hr of incubation at 35°C.

Mice were injected subcutaneously with 1 mg (50 mg/kg) of either ampicillin or streptomycin in 0.1 ml of saline. At the times of 15, 30, 60, 90, and 120 min after injection, approximately 1 ml of blood was obtained by retro-orbital bleeding. Each mouse was used for only one bleeding. Blood from 12 mice was pooled into three tubes for each time point of each antibiotic. Assays were carried out in triplicate in 15 cm diameter plates using 3 mm diameter holes. Wells were filled with 10 μl of serum. Antibiotic standards were prepared from reference ampicillin (Bristol) and streptomycin (Pfizer) powder diluted in normal mouse serum. Ampicillin was assayed in Penassay seed agar (Difco) using *Staphylococcus aureus* (American Type Culture Collection 6538) as the test organism. Incubation was carried out at 35°C for 18 hr. Detection levels were 1.2 to 10 μg/ml. Streptomycin was assayed in antibiotic assay medium No. 5 (Difco) using *Staphylococcus epidermidis* (from the National Institutes of Health) as the test organisms. Detection levels were 2 to 16 μg/ml.

CF-1 female mice were inoculated subcutaneously with approximately 10^3 viable *Y. pestis* organisms in 0.2 ml of saline. Treatment was started 24 or 48 hr after infection by subcutaneous injections of varying doses of antibiotics every 6 hr and continued for 3 days. Effective doses and durations of streptomycin were chosen from previous work and those of ampicillin were chosen to give blood antibacterial activity against *Y. pestis* comparable to that achieved with streptomycin. Mortality rates during 14 days of observation and the mean $\log_{10}$ of colony-forming units (CFU) per spleen at the end of antibiotic treatment were used as measurements of drug effect when compared to saline-treated control mice. All mice that died were autopsied and smears and cultures of the spleens were prepared. Five mice in each treatment group were sacrificed 6 hr after the last antibiotic injection for quantitative cultures of the spleen. The spleens were removed aseptically, washed twice with sterile water, and homogenized in 0.9% NaCl solution using glass homogenizers fitted with Teflon® pestles. Quantities of 0.1 ml of the homogenates and 10-

fold dilutions of the homogenates were spread onto nutrient agar plates, and colony counts were made after 24 hr of incubation at 35°C. Colonies were verified as being *Y. pestis* by specific bacteriophage lysis (phage obtained from Dr. C. R. Almeida, Garanhuns, Brazil). Additionally, to establish whether infections had occurred in culture-negative mice, serum of surviving mice was examined for the presence of antibodies against Fraction IA antigen of *Y. pestis* by a PHA, using antigen obtained from the Plague Branch of the Centers for Disease Control, Fort Collins, Colorado.

The three strains of *Y. pestis* were susceptible to ampicillin, penicillin, and streptomycin by the Kirby–Bauer method. The minimum inhibitory concentrations (MICs) of ampicillin against the strains used in this study were 3.3 μg/ml for *Y. pestis* strain 5, 0.1 μg/ml for strain 14, and 4.9 μg/ml for strain 18. The MICs of streptomycin against these strains were 0.3 μg/ml for strains 5 and 14 and 0.6 μg/ml for strain 18.

The serum concentrations of both antibiotics in mice following subcutaneous injections of 1 mg (50 mg/kg) showed rapid disappearance with half-lives of approximately 15–30 min. Streptomycin maintained higher blood concentrations during all sampling times and showed a slightly slower rate of elimination. Although serum levels of both antibiotics fell below detectable levels after 90 min, extrapolation of the decay curves indicated that streptomycin levels would remain greater than the median MIC of the strains of *Y. pestis* for more than 3 hr after injection, whereas ampicillin levels would remain above the median MIC for less than 1 hr.

In experimental infections with strain 18 of *Y. pestis*, graded doses of ampicillin and streptomycin were administered (Table 6.4). Mortality rates of mice were significantly reduced by ampicillin in doses less than 25 mg/kg and by streptomycin in doses less than 6.3 mg/kg ($p < 0.05$ by a Fisher Exact Test). In these doses, the mean $\log_{10}$ of CFU of *Y. pestis* per spleen in mice at the end of the antibiotic treatment period was reduced by more than 1000-fold (Table 6.4).

Large doses of antibiotics, 100 mg/kg of ampicillin and 50 mg/kg of streptomycin, which were respectively four and eight times greater than the least protective doses in the previous experiment, were administered to mice infected with three different strains of *Y. pestis* (Table 6.5). Mortality was reduced by both antibiotics in all experimental groups, but ampicillin was slightly less effective than streptomycin in reducing mortality. Both during and after treatment, the streptomycin-treated mice had better general appearances in regard to physical activity, body weight, and body hair than did the

TABLE 6.4
Responses of Murine Infections with *Yersinia pestis* Strain 18 to Ampicillin and Streptomycin[a]

Dose (mg/kg)	Mortality rate (No. dead/total)	Mean $\log_{10}$ CFU per spleen
Control (saline)	4/10	6.0
Ampicillin		
100	0/10	0
50	3/10	0
25	0/10	2.3
12.5	6/10	2.6
6.3	7/10	3.6
Streptomycin		
12.5	0/10	0
6.3	0/10	0
3.1	1/10	0
1.6	2/10	4.0
0.8	4/10	5.1

[a] Mice were infected by subcutaneous injection of 10^3 bacteria. Treatment was started 24 hr later by subcutaneous injection in a 0.1 ml volume and given every 6 hr for 3 days.

mice treated with ampicillin. Both drugs, however, rendered all spleens of infected mice sterile.

When sera of 50 surviving mice were tested for antibody titers against Fraction IA antigen of *Y. pestis,* 40 were positive with PHA titers $\geqslant 16$. This demonstrated that most of these surviving mice, which had been treated with

TABLE 6.5
Effects of Therapy with Ampicillin or Streptomycin in Experimental Murine *Yersinia pestis* Infection Produced by Three Different Strains of *Yersinia pestis*

	No. dead/total after 3 days of treatment			Mean $\log_{10}$ CFU per spleen after 3 days of treatment		
Treatment	*Y. pestis* Strain 5	*Y. pestis* Strain 14	*Y. pestis* Strain 18	*Y. pestis* Strain 5	*Y. pestis* Strain 14	*Y. pestis* Strain 18
Saline	5/10	4/10	8/10	4.1	5.4	6.8
Ampicillin	1/10	0/10	1/10	0	0	0
Streptomycin	0/10	0/10	0/10	0	0	0

[a] Treatment was ampicillin 100 mg/kg, streptomycin 50 mg/kg, or saline given subcutaneously every 6 hr for 3 days starting 2 days after inoculation with 10^3 bacteria.

an antibiotic, had recovered from active infections rather than having had their infections prevented entirely by the antibiotic treatment.

These results demonstrated that ampicillin prevents lethality in experimental murine plague infection and diminishes the bacterial burden in the spleen. The relevance of these findings to human plague is strengthened by the fact that the three strains of *Y. pestis* tested in this study were isolated from cases of human plague. These strains showed a median MIC of ampicillin of 3.3 μg/ml, and other strains tested recently from South Africa and Vietnam were also susceptible to ampicillin. All three strains were highly virulent in mice, producing lethal infections in most mice 8 days after subcutaneous infections with about 10^3 bacteria. Furthermore, treatment was started from 24–48 hours after inoculation, an adequate amount of time for bacteria to proliferate enough to cause serological responses to Fraction IA antigen of *Y. pestis*. Thus the therapy given in this study caused recovery from infections which would have been fatal to the mice.

In the dose ranges used in this study, ampicillin was slightly less effective than comparable doses of streptomycin in reducing mortality. The reason for the superiority of streptomycin in this model may be, in part, the longer half-life of streptomycin in blood after parenteral injection and the lower MICs of these strains to streptomycin. These findings suggest, nevertheless, that large doses of ampicillin given to patients with plague may be curative and that ampicillin deserves consideration as a less toxic alternative to streptomycin in the treatment of plague.

6.3.2. Supportive Therapy

Most patients with plague are febrile with constitutional symptoms including nausea and vomiting. Hypotension and dehydration are common. Therefore, intravenous 0.9% NaCl solution should be given to most patients for the first few days and until clinical improvement occurs. Patients in shock will require additional quantities of fluid with hemodynamic monitoring and the judicious use of epinephrine or dopamine. There is no evidence that corticosteroids or heparin are beneficial. Although the buboes usually recede without need of local therapy, they occasionally enlarge or become fluctuant during the 1st week of treatment, requiring incision and drainage. The fluid should be cultured to look for evidence of superinfection with other bacteria, but this material is usually sterile.

6.4. TREATMENT OF *YERSINIA* INFECTIONS

6.4.1. Antibiotic Therapy

Intestinal infection with *Y. enterocolitica* is usually self-limited and has been diagnosed so rarely that it is impossible at this time to assess the benefits of antibiotic treatment. In severe cases, especially in suspected extraintestinal infection, it is reasonable to use an antibiotic that is active against the particular strain of *Y. enterocolitica* isolated from a patient. Most isolates are suspectible to streptomycin, gentamicin, tetracycline, chloramphenicol, and trimethoprim–sulfamethoxazole; most isolates are resistant to the penicillins, certain cephalosporin antibiotics, and erythromycin.(61) The new 6-amidinopenicillanic acid antibiotic, mecillinam, was shown to be active against 48 strains of *Y. enterocolitica,* which were mostly resistant to ampicillin.(62) Thus, mecillinam may be a useful alternative to other drugs, especially in the setting of renal failure when aminoglycosides and trimethoprim–sulfamethoxazole are less advisable.

The new third-generation cephalosporin drug cefotaxime and the new monocyclic beta-lactam drug azthreonam were both active against five strains of *Y. enterocolitica.*(63) In France, Dabernat and Delmas(64) tested 22 strains of *Y. enterocolitica* also for susceptibility to the newer beta-lactam antibiotics. Those antibiotics that were most active *in vitro* with MICs of less than 1 μg/ml against half of the tested strains were mezlocillin, cefamandole, cefuroxime, cefotaxime, moxalactam, and ceftriaxone. Similarly, Goldstein *et al.*(65) found that cefotaxime, moxalactam, and gentamicin were the most active antibiotics against 14 strains of *Y. enterocolitica*. Although clinical studies of treating patients with these antibiotics have not been carried out, these results of *in-vitro* susceptibility suggest that the new cephalosporins may be the preferred antibiotics when patients with suspected disseminated infections with *Y. enterocolitica* require treatment.

Cornelis and co-workers(66) have identified plasmids of *Y. enterocolitica* that carry multiple antibiotic resistance. They found two different plasmids; one carried resistance to chloramphenicol, streptomycin, sulfonamide, and tetracycline and the other carried resistance to the same drugs except that kanamycin was substituted for tetracycline. Both plasmids could be transferred to *E. coli* K12 and to *Salmonella java*.

The penicillin resistance of *Y. entercolitica* was shown by Cornelis and Abraham(67,68) to be attributed to beta-lactamases. Two different enzymes were distinct by molecular weight, enzymatic range, and susceptibility to inhibition by cloxacillin. Gaspar and Soriano[69] tested the beta-lactamase inhibitor clavulanic acid and found that it had only a minimal action on 83 strains of *Y. enterocolitica*. They concluded that *Y. enterocolitica* produces a cephalosporinase rather than penicillinase.

When Kanazawa and Kuramata[70] compared 19 strains of *Y. pseudotuberculosis* with 40 strains of *Y. enterocolitica,* they found that the *Y. pseudotuberculosis* strains were uniformly susceptible to penicillin with MICs ranging from 0.05–0.8 μg/ml, whereas the *Y. enterocolitica* strains were resistant to no less than 12.5 μg/ml. Accordingly, all strains of *Y. pseudotuberculosis* did not produce beta-lactamase. These results suggest that serious extraintestinal *Y. pseudotuberculosis* infections can be treated with penicillin G.

6.4.2. Avoidance of Unnecessary Surgery

An aspect of diagnosis that is important to the treatment of *Yersinia* infections is to suspect the diagnosis in patients with severe abdominal pain in order to avoid unnecessary surgery for appendicitis. For this purpose, the recognition that early fever accompanies *Y. enterocolitica* infection may be helpful, as is epidemiological information pertaining to outbreaks in the community.

REFERENCES

1. T. Butler, A. A. F. Mahmoud, and K. S. Warren, Algorithms in the diagnosis and management of exotic diseases XXV. Plague, *J. Infect. Dis.* **136**:317–320 (1977).
2. W. J. Martin and J. A. Washington, Enterobacteriaceae, in *Manual of Clinical Microbiology,* Third Edition (E. H. Lennette, A. Balows, W. J. Hausler, and J. P. Truant, eds.), American Society of Microbiologists, Washington, D.C., pp.195–219 (1980).
3. M. P. Nunes and I. Suassuna, Bacteriophage specificity in the identification of *Yersinia pestis* as compared with other Enterobacteriaceae, *Rev. Bras. Pesqui. Med. Biol.* **11**:359–363 (1978).
4. M. J. Surgalla, E. D. Beesley, and J. M. Albizo, Practical applications of new laboratory methods for plague investigations, *Bull. W.H.O.* **42**:993–997 (1970).
5. T. J. Quan, J. J. Vanderlinden, and K. R. Tsuchiya, Evaluation of a qualitative isocitrate lyase assay for rapid presumptive identification of *Yersinia pestis* cultures, *J. Clin. Microbiol.* **15**:1178–1179 (1982).
6. T. H. Chen and S. S. Elberg, Scanning electron microscopic study of virulent *Yersinia pestis* and *Yersinia pseudotuberculosis* type I, *Infect. Immun.* **15**:972–977 (1977).

7. J. E. Williams, D. N. Harrison, T. J. Quan, J. L. Mullins, A. M. Barnes, and D. C. Cavanaugh, Atypical plague bacilli isolated from rodents, fleas, and man, *Am. J. Public Health* **68**:262–264 (1978).
8. B. W. Hudson, T. J. Quan, V. R. Sites, and J. D. Marshall, An electrophoretic and bacteriologic study of *Yersinia pestis* isolates from Central Java, Asia, and the Western hemisphere, *Am. J. Trop. Med. Hyg.* **22**:642–653 (1973).
9. B. W. Hudson and T. J. Quan, Electrophoretic studies of the yersiniae, *Am. J. Trop. Med. Hyg.* **24**:968–973 (1975).
10. B. W. Hudson, T. J. Quan, and R. E. Bailey, Electrophoretic studies of the geographic distribution of *Yersinia pestis* protein variants, *Int. J. Syst. Bacteriol.* **26**:1–16 (1976).
11. D. C. Cavanaugh, P. J. Deoras, D. H. Hunter, J. D. Marshall, D. V. Quy, J. H. Rust, S. Purnaveja, and P. E. Winter, Some observations on the necessity for serological testing of rodent sera for *Pasteurella pestis* antibody in a plague control programme, *Bull. W.H.O.* **42**:451–459 (1970).
12. E. E. Baker, H. Sommer, L. E. Foster, E. Meyer, and K. F. Meyer, Studies on immunization against plague I. The isolation and characterization of the soluble antigen of *Pasteurella pestis, J. Immunol.* **68**:131–145 (1952).
13. World Health Organization Expert Committee on Plague, Fourth Report, *W.H.O. Tech. Rep. Ser.* **447**:23–25 (1970).
14. S. Suzuki, Y. Chikasato, and S. Hotta, Studies on antiplague haemagglutinating antibodies, *Bull. W.H.O.* **51**:237–243 (1974).
15. S. Suzuki, H. Sakakibara, and S. Hotta, Latex agglutination tests for measurement of antiplague antibodies, *J. Clin. Microbiol.* **6**:332–336 (1977).
16. D. C. Cavanaugh, M. K. Fortier, D. M. Robinson, J. E. Williams, and J. H. Rust, Application of the ELISA technique to the problems in the serologic diagnosis of plague, *Bull. Pan Am. Health Organ.* **13**:399–402 (1979).
17. B. W. Hudson, K. Wolff, and T. Butler, The use of solid-phase radioimmunoassay techniques for serodiagnosis of human plague infection, *Bull. Pan Am. Health Organ.* **14**(3):244–250 (1980).
18. E. J. Bottone (ed.), *Yersinia enterocolitica,* CRC Press, Boca Raton, Florida, 224 p. (1981).
18a. G. Wauters, Contribution à l'étude de *Yersinia enterocolitica,* Ph.D. thesis, Catholic University, Vander, Louvain, Belgium (1970).
19. H. Bercovier, J. M. Alonso, Z. N. Bentaiba, J. Brault, and H. H. Mollaret, Contribution to the definition and the taxonomy of *Yersinia enterocolitica, Contrib. Microbiol. Immunol.* **5**:12–22 (1979).
20. D. J. Brenner, A. G. Steigerwalt, D. P. Falcao, R. E. Weaver, and G. R. Fanning, Characterization of *Yersinia enterocolitica* and *Y. pseudotuberculosis* by deoxyribonucleic acid hybridization and by biochemical reactions, *Int. J. Syst. Bacteriol.* **23**:205–216 (1976).
21. D. J. Brenner, Speciation in *Yersinia, Contrib. Microbiol. Immunol.* **5**:33–43 (1979).
22. E. J. Bottone, B. Chester, M. S. Malowany, and J. Allerhand, Unusual *Yersinia enterocolitica* isolates not associated with mesentery lymphadenitis, *Appl. Microbiol.* **27**:858–861 (1974).
23. B. Chester, G. Stotzky, E. J. Bottone, M. S. Malowany, and J. Allerhand, *Yersinia enterocolitica:* Biochemical, serological, and gas-liquid chromatographic characterization of rhamnose-, raffinose-, melibiose-, and citrate-utilizing strains, *J. Clin. Microbiol.* **6**:461–468 (1977).
24. P. M. Baker and J. J. Farmer, New bacteriophage typing system for *Yersinia enterocolitica, Yersinia kristensenii, Yersinia frederiksenii,* and *Yersinia intermedia:* Correlation with serotyping, biotyping,and antibiotic susceptibility, *J. Clin. Microbiol.* **15**:491–502 (1982).

25. E. J. Bottone, K. K. Sandhu, and M. A. Pisano, *Yersinia intermedia:* Temperature-dependent bacteriocin production, *J. Clin. Microbiol.* **10:**433–436 (1979).
26. G. Cornelis, R. K. J. Luke, and M. H. Richmond, Fermentation of raffinose by lactose-fermenting strains of *Yersinia enterocolitica* and sucrose-fermenting strains of *Escherichia coli, J. Clin. Microbiol.* **7:**180–183 (1978).
27. M. Tsubokura, K. Otsuki, I. Shimohira, and H. Yamamoto, Production of indirect hemolysin by *Yersinia enterocolitica* and its properties, *Infect. Immun.* **25:**939–942 (1979).
28. C. Calvo, J. Brault, J. M. Alonso, and H. H. Mollaret, New waterborne bacteriophages active on *Yersinia enterocolitica, Appl. Envir. Microbiol.* **42:**35–38 (1981).
29. A. K. Highsmith, J. C. Feeley, and G. K. Morris, *Yersinia enterocolitica:* A review of the bacterium and recommended laboratory methodology, *Health Lab. Sci.* **14:**253–260 (1977).
30. B. Nilehn, Bacteriological studies on 80 strains of *Yersinia enterocolitica* of human origin, *Symp. Ser. Immunobiol. Stand.* **9:**327–336 (1968).
31. B. Nilehn, Studies on *Yersinia enterocolitica:* Growth on various solid media at 37°C and 25°C, *Acta Pathol. Microbiol. Scand.* **77:**685–697 (1969).
32. C. H. Pai, S. Sorger, L. Lafleur, L. Lackman, and M. I. Marks, Efficacy of cold enrichment techniques for recovery of *Yersinia enterocolitica* from human stools, *J. Clin. Microbiol.* **9:**712–715 (1979).
33. A. Weissfeld and A. C. Sonnenwirth, *Yersinia*—a Canadian organism? *J. Pediatr.* **98:**504–505 (1981).
34. M. V. Dudley and E. B. Shotts, Medium for isolation of *Yersinia enterocolitica, J. Clin. Microbiol.* **10:**180–183 (1979).
35. J. Eiss, Selective culturing of *Yersinia enterocolitica* at low temperature, *Scand. J. Infect. Dis.* **7:**249–251 (1975).
36. A. S. Weissfeld and A. C. Sonnenwirth, *Yersinia enterocolitica* in adults with gastrointestinal disturbances: Need for cold enrichment, *J. Clin. Microbiol.* **11:**196–197 (1980).
37. J. R. Greenwood, S. M. Flanigan, M. J. Pickett, and W. J. Martin, Clinical isolation of *Yersinia enterocolitica:* Cold temperature enrichment, *J. Clin. Microbiol.* **2:**559–560 (1975).
38. A. S. Weissfeld and A. C. Sonnenwirth, Rapid isolation of *Yersinia* spp. from feces, *J. Clin. Microbiol.* **15:**508–510 (1982).
39. D. A. Schiemann, Synthesis of a selective medium for *Yersinia enterocolitica, Can. J. Microbiol.* **25:**1298–1304 (1979).
40. J. H. Bowen and S. D. Kominos, Evaluation of a pectin agar medium for isolation of *Yersinia enterocolitica* within 48 hours, *Am J. Clin. Pathol.* **72:**586–590 (1979).
41. T. D. Bartley, T. J. Quan, M. T. Collins, and S. M. Morrison, Membrane filter technique for the isolation of *Yersinia enterocolitica, Appl. Environ. Microbiol.* **43:**829–834 (1982).
42. D. A. Schiemann, Development of a two-step enrichment procedure for recovery of *Yersinia enterocolitica* from food, *Appl. Environ. Microbiol.* **43:**14–27 (1982).
42a. S. Winblad, B. Nilehn, and N. H. Sternby, *Yersinia enterocolitica* (*Pasteurella* X) in human enteric infection, *Br. Med. J.* **2:**1363–1366 (1966).
43. I. D. Ricciardi, A. D. Pearson, W. G. Suckling, and C. Klein, A microagglutination test for *Yersinia enterocolitica* infection: Recognition of multiple serotypes in experiments with stained suspensions of serotype O:5,27, *J. Med. Microbiol.* **11:**359–364 (1978).
44. K. Granfors, Measurement of immunoglobulin M (IgM), IgG, and IgA antibodies against *Yersinia enterocolitica* by enzyme-linked immunosorbent assay: Persistence of serum antibodies during disease, *J. Clin. Microbiol.* **9:**336–341 (1979).
45. M. Gripenberg, A. Nissinen, E. Vaisanen, and E. Linder, Demonstration of antibodies against *Yersinia enterocolitica* lipopolysaccharide in human sera by enzyme-linked immunosorbent assay, *J. Clin. Microbiol.* **10:**279–284 (1979).

46. S. Lang, H. Gunnarsson, P. Larsson, and H. Nygren, Diffusion-in-gel enzyme linked immunosorbent assay (DIG-ELISA) for detection of antibodies to *Yersinia enterocolitica, Acta Pathol. Microbiol. Scand. Sect. B* **89:**63–66 (1981).
47. K. Granfors, M. K. Viljanen, P. Ahvonen, and P. Toivanen, Measurement of IgM and IgG antibodies to *Yersinia* by solid-phase radioimmunoassay, *J. Infect. Dis.* **138:**232–236 (1978).
48. J. A. Maeland and A. Digranes, Common enterobacterial antigen in *Yersinia enterocolitica, Acta Pathol. Microbiol. Scand. Sect. B* **83:**382–386 (1975).
49. J. A. Maeland and A. Digranes, Human serum antibodies against heat-stable antigens from *Yersinia enterocolitica, Acta Pathol. Microbiol. Scand. Sect. B* **83:**451–456 (1975).
50. P. Ahvonen, E. Jansson, and K. Aho, Marked cross-agglutination between *Brucellae* and a subtype of *Yersinia enterocolitica, Acta Pathol. Microbiol. Scand.* **75:**291–295 (1969).
51. B. Hurvell, Serological cross-reactions between different *Brucella* species and *Yersinia enterocolitica, Acta Pathol. Microbiol. Scand. Sect. B* **81:**105–112 (1973).
52. B. Hurvell, Differentiation of cross-reacting antibodies against *Brucella abortus* and *Yersinia enterocolitica* by electroimmunoassay, *Acta Vet. Scand.* **16:**318–320 (1975).
53. B. Hurvell and A. A. Lindberg, Serological cross-reactions between different *Brucella* species and *Yersinia enterocolitica, Acta Pathol. Microbiol. Scand. Sect. B* **81:**113–119 (1973).
54. M. Schlesinger, S. Pollak, and P. A. Vardy, Cross-antigenicity between *Yersinia* and *Rickettsia, Isr. J. Med. Sci.* **15:**612–613 (1979).
55. K. Bech, J. H. Larsen, J. M. Hansen, and J. Nerup, *Yersinia enterocolitica* infection and thyroid disorders, *Lancet* **2:**951–952 (1974).
56. L. Shenkman and E. J. Bottone, Antibodies to *Yersinia enterocolitica* in thyroid disease, *Ann. Intern. Med.* **85:**735–739 (1976).
57. M. T. Reynolds, C. T. Keane, G. H. Tomkin, J. C. Roberts, T. J. Lenehan, and N. S. Mair, Antibodies to *Yersinia enterocolitica* serotype 3 in thyroid disease, *Br. Med. J.* **2:**400–401 (1978).
58. K. F. Meyer, S. F. Quan, F. R. McCrumb, and A. Larson, Effective treatment of plague, *Ann. N. Y. Acad. Sci.* **55:**1228–1274 (1952).
59. F. R. McCrumb, S. Mercier, J. Robic, M. Bouillat, J. E. Smadel, T. E. Woodward, and K. Goodner, Chloramphenicol and terramycin in the treatment of pneumonic plague, *Am. J. Med.* **14:**284–293 (1953).
60. N. V. Ai, N. D. Hanh, P. V. Dien, and N. V. Le, Effets in vitro and in vivo du trimethoprime–sulfamethoxazole sur *Yersinia pestis, Bull. Soc. Pathol. Exot.* **65:**759–765 (1972)).

60a. *Morbidity and Mortality Weekly Report* **24:**277 (1975).

61. S. Hammerberg, S. Sorger, and M. I. Marks, Antimicrobial susceptibilities of *Yersinia enterocolitica* Biotype 4, serotype O:3, *Antimicrob. Agents Chemother.* **11:**566–568 (1977).
62. I. Juhlin and S. Winblad, Susceptibility to mecillinam and other antibiotics of 28 O-serotypes of *Yersinia enterocolitica. J. Antibicrob. Chemother.* **8:**291–297 (1981).
63. H. C. Neu and P. Labtharikul, Antibacterial activity of a monocyclic beta-lactam SQ 26,776, *J. Antibicrob. Chemo. Suppl. E* 111–122 (1981).
64. H. J. Dabernat and C. Delmas, Comparative activity of cefotaxime and selected beta-lactam antibiotics against *Hemophilus influenzae* and aerobic gram-negative bacilli, *Rev. Infect. Dis.* **4**(Suppl.)**:**S401–S405 (1982).
65. E. J. C. Goldstein, C. E. Cherubin, M. L. Corrado, and M. F. Sierra, Comparative susceptibility of *Yersinia enterocolitica, Eikenella corrodens,* and penicillin-susceptible *Streptococcus pneumoniae* to beta-lactam and alternative antibicrobial agents, *Rev. Infect. Dis.* **4**(Suppl.)**:**S406–S410 (1982).

66. G. Cornelis, G. Wauters, and G. Bruynoghe, Resistances transferables chez des souches sauvages de *Yersinia enterocolitica, Ann. Microbiol.* **124:**299–209 (1973).
67. G. Cornelis and E. P. Abraham, Beta-lactamases from *Yersinia enterocolitica, J. Gen. Microbiol.* **87:**273–284 (1975).
68. G. Cornelis, Distribution of beta-lactamases A and B in some groups of *Yersinia enterocolitica* and their role in resistance, *J. Gen. Microbiol.* **91:**391–402 (1975).
69. M. C. Gaspar and F. Soriano, Susceptibility of *Yersinia enterocolitica* to eight beta-lactam antibiotics and clavulanic acid, *J. Antibicrob. Chemother.* **8:**161–164 (1981).
70. Y. Kanazawa and T. Kuramata, Difference in susceptibility to benzylpenicillin between *Yersinia enterocolitica* and *Yersinia pseudotuberculosis, Jpn. J. Microbiol.* **18:**483–485 (1974).

7

Prevention and Control

The epidemic and fatal nature of plague infection has stimulated enormous efforts by public health workers to seek effective control measures against this disease. Plague is today one of only four internationally quarantinable diseases, along with cholera, smallpox, and yellow fever. Although plague is relatively well controlled today, being restricted in human cases to less than 1000 per year in all countries except Vietnam and Burma, the disease has the potential for rapid expansion from the endemic foci that exist in many countries. Public health workers in all such countries, as well as the World Health Organization (WHO), keep constant vigilance over the plague incidence in the world, ever fearful that new outbreaks will occur that will be difficult to control.

The control of the other *Yersinia* infections is a subject that is in its infancy when compared to plague. Thus, the other diseases will be considered separately.

7.1. CONTROL OF PLAGUE

There are many possible approaches to the control of plague, and the best one for each situation will be determined by the particular place, extent of the epidemic, and the available personnel and facilities. The early steps in control require accurate information on diagnosis of human cases. Patients must be seen by qualified medical workers and bubo aspirates must be obtained for smears and cultures and sera obtained for serology. After the presence of *Yersinia pestis* infection has been established as the cause of an epidemic, treatment with the antibiotics streptomycin or tetracycline should be provided in order to diminish human mortality. Prophylactic antibiotic treatment with streptomycin or tetracycline for 2 days should be given to family contacts and other intimate contacts of patients with suspected pneumonic plague to prevent spread of the disease by the airborne route.

After the medical attention has been given personally to cases and their contacts, epidemiologic surveillance of the area must be carried out to assess the geographic regions affected, the time of infection in each area, the ages and sexes of involved persons, the mortality rates, and evidences of human contacts with rodents. Because plague is a zoonotic infection, involving primarily rodents and their fleas, it is essential to have experienced public health workers who are mammalogists or entomologists or other persons with similar backgrounds with field work. Evidence of epizootic plague must be sought by obtaining information from local people about rodent die-offs, by autopsies of dead rodents for culture of the blood, spleen, and liver, and by trapping live rodents which will be observed in captivity for mortality, autopsy, and be used for serological surveillance.

With this epidemiological information, it is possible to formulate a rational control plan. Good control plans usually place varying emphasis on rodent control by trapping or rodenticide use, vector control by insecticide use, education of people to avoid contact with rodents, rat-proofing of houses, and vaccination of high-risk persons. Table 7.1 lists eight different strategies for the control of plague. The priorities for implementing each of these strategies will depend on the local assessment of any given outbreak and on the availability of materials and personnel. The effectiveness of the various strategies will be further discussed in this chapter.

In 1979, the WHO convened a consultative group to make recommendations about plague control. The views of this informal consultation have been published and will be presented in part[(1)]:

> When bubonic plague cases or outbreaks occur, the first control measures should be carried out against the flea population in the affected locality, followed immediately by control of rodents. Limited bubonic plague episodes can be ended easily if early specific treatment of patients is initiated and if the rodent flea population in the affected area is effectively controlled. Flea control consists of the proper application of an effective insecticide. Regular testing for insecticide resistance should be carried out on flea populations in plague-potential areas. WHO provides a standardized and reliable test kit that should be used for this

TABLE 7.1
Strategies for the Control of Plague and the Effectiveness of These Strategies

Strategy	Effectiveness
Antibiotic treatment of cases	Effective in reducing human mortality, potentially effective to prevent rare pneumonic transmission to other persons, no effect on natural reservoirs
Flea control by insecticide use	Unknown, believed to be effective
Rodent control by poisoning and trapping	Effective in urban plague
Antibiotic prophylaxis for persons in contact with suspected cases of pneumonic plague	Untested but probably effective
Quarantine of human cases	Probably not of use if antibiotic is used
Ship inspection in ports	Effective
Vaccines	Indirect evidence for effectiveness in preventing human cases, no effect on natural reservoirs and transmission
Education of people to avoid contact with rodents, prevent rodent harborage, and to control fleas on pets	Unknown

purpose. Rodent control, following flea control, is carried out during or after any plague outbreak in humans. Rodents, particularly those living in houses, are best controlled by poisoning. When the extremely contagious pulmonary plague cases occur, immediate isolation and treatment of the patient and prophylactic treatment (with antibiotics for at least seven days) of all known contacts are essential to prevent further spread.

Surveillance and Control at the National Level. Wherever there is a history of past plague infection, there exists the possibility that infected fleas or rodents could be exported, or that persons unknowingly infected with plague could introduce plague into new areas. Good surveillance and control are indispensable. The meeting recommended that the public health services of each country concerned be prepared to carry out surveillance and emergency control of plague, using personnel specially trained for these purposes.

Staff operating in plague foci must be capable of identifying the clinical symptoms of plague and the overt signs of plague in animal populations. They should be supported at the national or regional level by a specialized laboratory staffed with an epidemiologist, a bacteriologist, and a field biologist, each with assistants. The staff would be responsible for (1) laboratory diagnosis of human plague; (2) early detection of suspected cases and hospitalization of patients; (3) control over the work carried out in plague hospitals and isolation wards; (4) prophylaxis of contacts of human cases; (5) rodent and flea control, including pesticide susceptibility studies; and (6) health education.

The specialized plague team should be equipped with all necessary facilities for its activities and with land and emergency air transport. There should be ongoing education of the team at a high level.

Development of a Phased Plague Surveillance and Control Program. Each country has a different health system and different resources. The meeting developed a four-phase program, graduated in its degree of sophistication and in the demands it makes on the health system. Phases I and II comprise the most basic and immediate steps to be taken in the event of a plague outbreak in humans; Phases III and IV include measures to be taken for predictive surveillance and preventive control, research and development, and environmental management. [Table 7.2 gives an outlined summary of the four phases and their components.]

TABLE 7.2
Four Phases of Plague Control Program Suggested by World Health Organization Informal Consultation[1]

Phase I: Case recognition and medical intervention

Clinical diagnosis of *Y. pestis* is made; treatment of the patient(s) is initiated; the bacillus is isolated and tentatively identified, then confirmed at a regional or central laboratory.

Preliminary epidemiological investigation is carried out and the potential animal or human sources of infection discovered.

Case contacts are observed and treated when necessary.

Health authorities and the medical community and public must be informed.

The utility of vaccination of select groups must be evaluated.

Phase II: Epidemiological/epizootiological investigation and emergency control

Specific sites at which infection was acquired are located, and the animal and vector species potentially involved are identified.

Vector and rodent populations in contact with people and potentially harmful to them are identified.

Ecological factors are taken into consideration for developing control strategies.

The geographical extent of the epidemic/epizootic is estimated by rapid surveys.

Emergency vector operations are initiated.

Phase III: Predictive surveillance and preventive control

Research is conducted to establish a predictive surveillance system and control criteria suited to the focus.

Preventive control strategies are developed based on surveillance data, landscape characteristics, and host/vector ecology.

Research to develop environmental control measures is implemented.

Continuing public information and health education on plague are provided.

Phase IV: Management

This phase involves continuing surveillance in plague enzootic and epizootic areas.

Preemptive control measure are undertaken on the basis of the predictive surveillance program.

Environmental management is used to maintain reduced populations of commensal and key wild rodent reservoir species.

There should be continuing community education and exchange of information among agencies and institutions concerned with plague research, surveillance, and control.

Research and development in the areas of plague diagnosis, microbiology, therapy, ecology, and control is continued.

International Cooperation

International Health Regulations. The International Health Regulations of 1969 give basic guidelines on the organization of plague surveillance. Constraints on international travellers are minimal, and plague vaccination is not required. Under these regulations, a health administration is required to keep itself informed about plague conditions by the regular examination of rodents and their ectoparasites. Any port, airport, or area which is infected or suspected of being infected with plague should be given particular attention. It is also stipulated that health authorities for each port and airport shall take all practicable measures to keep the installation free of rodents. WHO publishes a list of ports which must be equipped to issue deratting exemption certificates to ships and, where the deratting of ships is necessary, to carry out the procedure.

Notifications of cases and deaths and other relevant information received by WHO are reported to Member States in the WHO *Weekly Epidemiological Record,* which also publishes a summary of the plague situation in the world once a year. The automatic telex reply service of WHO is used for epidemiological information of special importance.

Reference, Research and Training Activities. The WHO Expert Committee on Plague in 1969 recommended the establishment of one or more reference centres for plague, whose function would be to provide technical cooperation to countries in the identification of *Y. pestis* and other *Yersinia* species, the identification of rodents and other mammals and of fleas and other ectoparasites, the production and maintenance of specific sera and antigens for distribution to national reference centres, the collection and analysis of epidemiological data on plague, and the training of personnel.

The WHO Collaborating Center for Reference and Research on Plague, established in 1973 in Stavropol, U.S.S.R., has been carrying out these functions and others, such as cooperative studies with other laboratories to evaluate the haemagglutination test. Other WHO activities include the organization of several traveling seminars in the field of plague and vector biology and control. (pp. 141–142)

7.1.1. Sentinel Animals for Plague Surveillance

A useful approach to the surveillance of plague in rodents has been to obtain blood from carnivores and measure antiplague antibodies. For this purpose, dogs were used in Vietnam and coyotes have been used in California.[(2)] Carnivores rarely develop illness after ingesting plague-infected rodents, but they develop self-limited infections with the appearance of telltale antibodies. Willeberg and co-workers correctly located areas of plague activity in California by using coyotes as sentinel animals.[(2)] The direct examination of rodent sera for antibodies also has been useful to detect areas of active or recent plague infection.[(3)] This method, however, is more expensive and time-consuming than the use of sentinel animals because it requires trapping and bleeding of many individual rodents at different times and in different places.

7.1.2. Effectiveness of Strategies for Plague Control

The effectiveness of plague vaccine is controversial and will be considered separately in the next section. The effectiveness of the other strategies in Table 7.1 is also difficult to judge, but some critical assessment of these efforts is necessary in order to make rational recommendations concerning their use. First of all, none of the control measures has been rigorously evaluated in the field by a controlled, randomized, and double-blinded trial to test effectiveness against a nonintervention or placebo alternative. Thus, none of the measures has been proven effective beyond any doubt. This uncertainty about effectiveness of control measures is further compounded by the complexity of natural variables that govern the propagation of plague in the environment. Many of these variables operate, fortunately, to limit the spread of plague. Some of these natural factors that control plague have been mentioned in Chapter 3 and include seasonal variation due to effects of temperature and humidity on fleas, die-off of the susceptible rodent populations, development of immunity in both human and rodent populations after exposure to plague bacilli, and alterations in the virulence of epidemic strains of *Y. pestis*.

Antibiotic treatment of human cases always must be given priority in an epidemic of plague because it is lifesaving. But the use of antibiotics in humans will have little, if any, impact on the spread of plague, owing to the usual route of infection from rodents to man. A potential benefit of antibiotic use in man could be the suppression of some cases of bubonic plague which would progress to pneumonic plague and become contagious by the airborne route. The progression of these infections would be aborted by antibiotic treatment, but pneumonic transmission of plague has been so rare in recent decades that this effect of antibiotics is impossible to evaluate at this time.

The use of insecticides in people's houses is usually given high priority during epidemics of plague. Insecticides are generally available and the application of insecticides is a visible activity of a plague control effort. Insecticides offer the promise of interrupting the final step of transmission of the infection from rodents to man. They could have a secondary benefit of interrupting transmission among rodent reservoirs, if they are dispensed widely enough to reach areas of rodent harborage. The limitations of insecticide use are also obvious and include the resistance of certain flea populations to insecticides, the difficulty of applying adequate amounts of insecticides to relevant areas to ensure that rodent fleas will be killed before they can bite humans, and the toxicity of insecticides for man. Some plague workers warn that rodenticide use without concomitant insecticide use will exacerbate a human plague outbreak by causing fleas to depart the dead rodents and have increased contact with man, but this phenomenon has never been verified in practice.

Rodent control is the least controversial measure that must be central in any plague control program. Rodents are the major reservoirs of plague infection and their central importance in plague epidemics cannot be ignored. Epidemics of plague always are accompanied by epizootics in the reservoir animals. Rat control in cities reportedly has produced dramatic results in stopping epidemics. Although rat control has not been tested for efficacy in controlled studies, the evidence would appear overwhelming that this approach is effective. It is logical that reduced numbers of susceptible animals will provide less opportunity for the infection to spread among animals and, thus, less chance for man to make contact with infected rodents and their fleas. In cities with large rat populations, there needs to be a well-publicized campaign to kill rats by rodenticides and by trapping, and to limit availability of rat food, e.g., by using metal garbage cans with tight-fitting lids. Houses should be modified to be rat-proof. In rural areas, where plague is enzootic, however, as in the United States, rodent control is not a feasible approach because rodents live in widespread, diverse habitats that cannot be selectively contaminated by poisons. Besides, rodent control in sylvatic foci might have undesirable environmental effects. Any attempt to eliminate a species of rodents from a geographical area would be challenged by environmental advocates. One real concern with sylvatic rodent control would be that other species of rodents might increase, as a result of eliminating plague reservoirs, and other zoonotic diseases such as salmonellosis, tularemia, and relapsing fever might increase in a given geographic area.

Recent work by Brooks *et al.*[(4)] in Burma has approached the problem of rat control. They showed that the bandicoot rat was more susceptible to brodifacoum and to difenacoum than to warfarin. They suggest that these anticoagulant drugs could be useful in the field but that drug resistance after periods of use could be overcome by using toxicant drugs like zinc phosphide and pyrinuron in alternation with the anticoagulants. The acute toxicant drug scilliroside was tested also in Burma against bandicoot rats and found to be effective.[5]

The quarantine of human cases of plague has almost no role in the control of plague today. The use of antibiotics renders patients with pneumonic plague noncontagious within minutes after treatment. Thus, quarantine measures would be useless. International quarantine is also practically irrelevant. The incubation period of plague is very short, usually less than 5 days and there are no long-term human carriers of plague infection that are a hazard to other persons. Therefore, the control of travelers from plague-infected areas will have little or no impact on the spread of plague. The transportation of rodents, however, on ships or other conveyances such as wagons and trains has been an important factor in the spread of plague infection during recent history. Shipping ports are still infested with rats in many areas of the world, and the constant vigilance of ships by health inspectors is necessary to prevent the dissemination of plague.

More recent recommendations to control plague have arisen from case–control studies in the United States.[5a] Persons with plague were shown to live in houses near places of rodent harborage. These places included old tires and other containers, and there was food available for the rodents. Persons with plague also were more likely to have pets with fleas, and the exchange of fleas between infected rodents and pets was considered to play a role in bringing plague to the people (see Chapter 3). Thus, it is reasonable to educate people in these plague-endemic areas to clear their yards of rodent harborage objects and rodent food. They should also control fleas on their household pets. The effectiveness of these suggested measures has not yet been measured.

7.1.3. Plague Vaccine: A Brief History

The development of plague vaccines originated in 1894 just after Yersin discovered the plague bacillus and Emile Roux urged him to develop an attenuated vaccine bacterium. Many different vaccine preparations, including both killed and live vaccine, have been used and tested. In recent years the late K. F. Meyer and his co-workers worked very productively to improve the safety and efficacy of plague vaccines.

The reader who is interested in the history of plague vaccines should refer to recent papers by Meyer and his colleagues.[6,7] The development of vaccines for man has taken two distinct pathways: the development of killed vaccines and the development of living attenuated vaccines. The killed vaccine gained greater use and the currently recommended vaccine in the United States, Plague Vaccine, U.S.P., is a killed preparation. The reasons for the ascendancy of the killed vaccine were its potentially better protective efficacy by virtue of its certain immunogenicity and its greater safety than the living vaccines, which carried the potential for reverting to a virulent form and causing damage.

The first killed vaccine was developed by Haffkine in Bombay, India, in 1897. This vaccine was injected subcutaneously and produced fever, localized swelling and erythema, and regional lymphadenopathy. Vaccinated persons were incapacitated for a day or two. These severe side effects led to the discontinuation of this approach in 1935. Although there was some evidence that the Haffkine vaccine was protective, some vaccinated individuals developed plague infections.

During World War II, renewed efforts to develop a safer killed plague vaccine were initiated by Meyer and his co-workers in San Francisco. They determined that formalin-killed cultures of fully virulent *Y. pestis* produced antibody responses that would suggest that they conferred protective immunity. Animal protection studies indicated that the vaccines were effective. The vaccines were given subcutaneously to human volunteers. When the number of injected bacteria did not exceed 2×10^9, the local and systemic reactions were not so severe as to preclude mass immunization. Vaccination with killed vaccine was carried out in American armed forces.

The presently available Plague Vaccine, U.S.P., emerged from these studies. It consists of an aqueous suspension of virulent *Y. pestis* (Indian isolate 195 P) grown on agar medium at 37°C for 48 hr. The organisms are harvested in saline and killed by adding formalin to a final concentration of 0.5%. Each milliliter contains 2×10^9 bacilli, which are stored in 0.5% phenol.

The efficacy of killed vaccines in preventing human plague has been claimed but never proven in a randomized field trial. Indirect evidence that killed vaccines are protective has been presented by Meyer,[(6)] who stated that no vaccinated Americans during World War II developed plague despite considerable exposure to infection in the field. During the Vietnam conflict, Cavanaugh *et al.*[(8)] pointed out that eight cases of plague were reported among a huge American military presence. The researchers estimated that this is only one case per million man years of exposure. Since all military personnel were required to be vaccinated, they argue that this fact suggests protective efficacy.

Furthermore, the investigators[8] documented a rise in antibody titers against Fraction I antigen of *Y. pestis* in patients hospitalized with murine typhus. Both murine typhus and plague were transmitted by rat fleas in Vietnam, and these data indicated that some persons developed dual infections. The asymptomatic nature of some of these plague infections also may argue indirectly for the efficacy of the plague vaccine.

The history of the live attenuated plague vaccines goes back to 1908 when Strong used a vaccine in Manila. Further testing was carried out by Girard and Robic in 1933 and by Otten in 1934 in Madagascar and in Indonesia, respectively. Most work has been done with the EV 76 strain of *Y. pestis,* which contains Fraction I and V and W antigens, but does not produce pigment on media that contain hemin. These vaccine strains are protective because they multiply and persist in the tissues, but cannot proliferate with sufficient rapidity to produce plague disease.

The side effects of live vaccines are similar to those of the killed vaccines. They can produce local reactions and systemic reactions that consist of fever, lymphadenopathy, headache, weakness, malaise, and skin sloughing or pustule formation. In general, the side effects associated with live vaccine use are more severe than with killed vaccines. Meyer *et al.*[7] noted that reactions of individuals vaccinated in Madagascar with EV 76 were severe, sometimes resulting in hospitalization of the vaccinees.

Another problem with the live vaccines has been wide variations in their immunogenicity and virulence. Strains have reportedly lost their immunogenic effects, perhaps because of mutation or plasmid loss. Meyer tested several EV vaccine strains and found that they did not provoke serologic responses in man that are associated with acquired immunity. In animal studies, the EV vaccines have not shown good protective immunity. Perhaps the most alarming feature of the avirulent live vaccines is the potential for reverting to virulent forms. Meyer indicated that the standard Girard EV 76 isolate could be enhanced in virulence by passage through rats and guinea pigs. A small dose of 2.2×10^3 organisms of EV 51f caused fatal infections in vervets.

The effectiveness of the living vaccines has been claimed but not proven. Vaccine use was considered to be highly effective in preventing plague in Indonesia and Madagascar because infection rates and mortality rates were reduced in vaccinated subjects. However, the unvaccinated subjects with higher infection and mortality rates were not randomized or given placebo-vaccine as proper controls need to be in a vaccine field trial. Thus, the effectiveness of live vaccines in man to prevent plague infection remains a controversial and clouded question.

7.1.4. Use of Plague Vaccine in Vietnam

Live plague vaccine was administered to more than ten million Vietnamese people between 1967 and 1969. A report by Liem and Jullien presented in Saigon in 1970 summarized their experience with vaccines.[9]

> In Vietnam, plague was recorded as occurring in 1898 in Nhatrang, in 1901 in Tonkin (North Vietnam) and in 1908 in Saigon. Since that time, it lingers under endemic form and tends to reappear during the hottest months preceding the rainy season. During the recent years, plague incidence has increased throughout the country. Mass vaccination, although with a questionable efficaciousness while used as a measure of plague control, has been however used generally as a prophylactic arm. Given the conditions of endemicity and the difficulties the application of general methods of systematic rodent control, the vaccination campaign in Vietnam has taken on a special importance.
>
> The first human vaccinations against plague were made by Haffkine in 1897 in Bombay with a killed vaccine and by Strong in Manila with a living vaccine in 1906. At the beginning of this century, in Vietnam, people utilized the killed vaccine from Pasteur Institute of Paris, and sent to Saigon by ship, for distribution to the whole Indochinese peninsula. It was only in 1938, after trial vaccinations had been carried out in Madagascar, that the plague vaccinal strain came to Pasteur Institute in Dalat where it was kept for the production of living vaccine. In consequence of the disturbances in the years 1945–47 and of the scarcity of transportation means, Pasteur Institute in Saigon had to ensure the production of vaccines, in order to meet the needs of civil and military health services.
>
> Therefore, for more than 30 years, Pasteur Institute in Vietnam has been manufacturing living plague vaccine, which is a suspension in normal saline solution of plague bacilli of one billion per millilitre. In general, it was before 1969 the only vaccine that could be made available to the civilian population. During the recent years, killed vaccines from foreign sources have been available too, and originate from either Haffkine Institute (India), or from Cutter Laboratory (U.S.).
>
> For the preparation of living vaccine at Pasteur Institute in Saigon, *Pasteurella pestis* EV 76 strain of Girard and Robic has been used; this strain was isolated in 1926 in Madagascar, its virulence being attenuated through successive subcultures in gelose during 5 years. This strain kept in Pasteur Institute of Paris is considered as the most appropriate for the production of living vaccine. It must be strictly controlled and kept in such a way to conserve all its initial character. Criteria of preservation and activity are those advocated by their authors, and based on anatomo-pathological lesions in guinea pigs. The strain is kept in a enriched peptone, maintained at a constant temperature of 4°C, with only one subculture per year, to conserve the antigenic characters of the germ.

Manufacture should be carried out conforming to the needs, and no security stock will be possible. The present capacity of production is approximately 100,000 doses per week and can be quadrupled in case of need. Given a population of approximately 17 millions the figures concerning the distribution and utilization of vaccines during these recent years are as follows:

	Distribution (doses)	Vaccination (No. of persons)
1967	3,800,000	2,743,333
1968	8,350,000	6,140,582
1969	8,150,000	4,428,201

It should be noted that, owing to logistical difficulties and to those met with in the storage of living vaccine, Pasteur Institute in Vietnam is thinking of collaterally assuming the production of killed plague vaccine. For this purpose, the technical collaboration of the World Health Organization has been requested for and the assignment of one consultant is expected. The primary advantage of killed vaccine resides in the fact that it presents logistical convenience and that the period of utilization is longer. Furthermore, less marked vaccinal reactions make its use more desirable in vaccination campaigns and more easily acceptable by the population. However, it presents operational difficulties occasioned by repeated injections given at short intervals; moreover, the immunity which it affords is considered as less constant and less lasting.

After the change of government in 1975 in Vietnam, the large effort to vaccinate the people underwent changes. Although complete information on plague in Vietnam after 1975 remains unavailable, it is known that human plague persisted as a health problem. Public health facilities were altered, medical supplies became scarce, and external collaborations ceased temporarily.

Despite the claims of vaccine efficacy in Vietnam, it appears that this massive effort to vaccinate over 10,000,000 people was futile. The reasons are the doubtful immunogenic potency of the live vaccine and the inherent limitations in using a vaccine in humans against a zoonotic infection. Plague was too seriously out of control in the rodents due to the wartime conditions, and the people were forced to live in proximity to the infected rats. Protecting man with vaccines, which may have themselves been ineffective, was cumbersome and could not reach all the people. Whether a better effort could have been made through more rodent control and insecticide use is a matter for speculation.

7.1.5. Recommended Use of Vaccines Today

There is only one commercially available plague vaccine being produced in the world today. This is Plague Vaccine, U.S.P., manufactured by Cutter Laboratories (Berkeley, California 94710 U.S.), and it contains the highly virulent Indian strain 195 P of *Y. pestis,* which is killed and preserved in formalin 0.4 ml/liter and phenol 5 ml/liter. During the Vietnam conflict of the 1960s and 1970s more than a million doses of this vaccine were given to U.S. servicemen. Despite the existence of this plague vaccine, vaccines should play little or no role in programs to control plague infection. The reasons for this diminished role of plague vaccine can be summarized as follows:

1. As plague is a zoonotic infection, with man being an accidental host who plays no role in the maintenance or propagation of the infection in nature, the vaccination of man can only prevent human infection but cannot have any impact on the animal reservoirs in nature.
2. Antibacterial immunity is short-lived. Revaccination is recommended every 6 months.
3. The expense and impracticality of vaccinating people in developing countries with limited health budgets and trained personnel should be apparent.

Furthermore, the efficacy of this vaccine has not been documented in a controlled vaccine field trial. The vaccine is intended to stimulate acquired immunity against plague. Although recurrent plague is very rare and this rarity of reinfection serves as the basis for the belief in the protective value of natural immunity as well as the vaccine, recurrent infections have been reported.

In Vietnam, Butler and Hudson[10] documented recurrent infections in 2 out of 82 patients with plague who were being tested for antiplague antibodies. Two of the 82 patients who were studied gave a history of previous plague infection 4 and 6 years, respectively, before their present illness. In both cases the previous positive bubo cultures for *Y. pestis* were documented in the records of the Pasteur Institute in Saigon, and one patient had had a convalescent passive hemagglutination (PHA) antibody titer of 1 : 64. The PHA antibody titers of both these patients were significantly elevated at the time of admission (Table 7.3). These high titers at the time of admission contrast with those of the remaining 80 patients, who did not have a history of previous infection and who did not have a titer greater than 1 : 16 on Day

TABLE 7.3
Recurrent *Yersinia pestis* Infections

Age (years)	Sex	Interval between infections (years)	Bubo culture	Log$_2$ PHA antibody titer to Fraction I antigen of *Y. pestis*			
				Admission		Convalescence	
				Log$_2$ titer	Day of illness	Log$_2$ titer	Day of illness
10	F	4	Negative	6	1	3	8
70	F	6	Positive	8	3	6	8

1 of illness or greater than 1 : 32 on Day 3 of illness. Both patients with a recurrent infection showed a significant decrease in PHA antibody titer (8-fold and 4-fold, respectively) when retested during convalescence. None of the other 45 patients, in whom paired sera were examined, showed a decrease in titer. In 40 of these patients, a four-fold or greater increase in titer occurred between the time of admission and during convalescence, and in five patients no significant change occurred. Both patients with recurrent infection were treated with streptomycin and recovered satisfactorily. Their illnesses were no less severe than those of other patients, and their response to therapy was no more rapid than that of the other patients.

The Advisory Committee of Immunization Practices in the United States issued its recommendations in 1982 for the use of the plague vaccine.[11] Because plague is rare in most parts of the world today, there is no need to vaccinate persons except those at exceptionally high risk. For example, field workers like ecologists, geologists, archeologists, Peace Corps volunteers, or agricultural advisors who are planning to work in an area that is known to have rodent plague should be considered to receive the vaccine. Similarly, laboratory workers who will handle plague cultures or plague-infected animals should be immunized. Medical workers and public health workers who are dealing with patients with plague or who are investigating plague outbreaks are at increased risk of developing infection and should consider receiving immunization. Routine immunization is not advised for travelers who are going to endemic areas or for residents of these areas.

The plague vaccine is believed to provide protection against fleaborne plague but might not give protection against airborne pneumonic plague.

Therefore, all persons exposed to patients with suspected pneumonic plague should receive antibiotic prophylaxis, regardless of their immunization status.

All injections of the Plague Vaccine, U.S.P., are given intramuscularly. Adults and children over 10 years should receive a primary series of 1.0 ml, followed by a second dose of 0.2 ml 4 weeks later. A third dose of 0.2 ml is given 6 months after the first dose. In cases of continuing exposure, booster doses of 0.2 ml are given every 6 months up to three times. Thereafter, booster doses can be given at 1- or 2-year intervals. Reduced dosage volumes are recommended for children.[(11)]

Vaccination may result in side effects of fever, headache, malaise, lymphadenopathy, and erythema and induration at the injection site. These reactions are more common after repeated injections. Sterile abscesses rarely occur. Urticarial and asthmatic reactions have been reported rarely. The vaccine should not be given to persons with known hypersensitivity to beef protein, soya, casein, or phenol. Persons with a history of severe local or systemic reactions to plague vaccine should not be revaccinated. Pregnant women should not be vaccinated because of the potential ability of vaccines to produce abortions or fetal abnormalities.

7.1.6. Newer Approaches to Vaccination

Newer approaches to vaccination against plague have been investigated in recent years. The immunity that is conferred by parenteral vaccination has been measured by antibody responses against Fraction I antigen of *Y. pestis*. Although serum antibody titers may reflect the degree of protective immunity conferred by a vaccine, there is no evidence that immunity results directly from these circulating antibodies. Williams and Cavanaugh[(12)] have reported that levels of antibody against Fraction I antigen in rats are less protective against intranasal challenge with *Y. pestis* than against subcutaneous challenge. This finding suggests that immunity against plague pneumonia that is acquired by inhalation of an aerosol may be mediated by local mucosal immunity which is functional on the epithelial surfaces of the tracheobronchial tree. Circulating antibodies may or may not reflect the activity of the mucosal immunity. Recent work on mucosal immunity has indicated that the traffic patterns of lymphocytes involve pathways that link the expressions of mucosal immunity in the intestine, lung, and breast. Thus, immunization of the intestinal mucosa will result in local immunity in the lung and breast milk as well as in the intestine. Chen *et al.*[13] have shown that the oral administration of a live vaccine strain of *Y. pestis* to vervets resulted in immune protection against pneumonic plague which was induced by inhalation challenge. Thus, the direct vaccination of mucosal surfaces may be a useful future direction in plague immunology.

A promising new approach is to seek cross-protective immunity against plague by using vaccines that consist of different bacteria. Alonso *et al.*[14] have shown that mice that are convalescing from infection with *Yersinia enterocolitica* serotype O:3 are resistant to *Y. pestis* infection. Only when *Y. enterocolitica* was grown at 25°C was good protection observed. Subculturing *Y. enterocolitica* at 37°C led to decreased cross-protection, as well as to decreased survival in mice and to loss of the property of autoagglutination. Mice that were immunized with *Y. enterocolitica* displayed footpad swelling when injected with dead *Y. pestis,* indicating a cross-reaction of delayed hypersensitivity.

Other new approaches to our understanding of plague immunity have originated from new knowledge of cellular immunity. Although most attention has been focused on humoral immunity, the role of host cells in defending against plague has been recognized for a long time. Jewetz and Meyer in 1944 summarized some of the relationships between serum immune factors and cellular functions in plague immunity[15]:

1. The serum, plasma, or other body fluids of animals that are immune to plague infection are unable to destroy or lyse *Y. pestis* organisms *in vitro* and *in vivo* in the absence of phagocytic cells.
2. Whole blood of plague-immune animals can destroy a much greater number of plague bacilli than blood of normal animals. This higher specific activity is primarily inherent in the plasma, not in the cells.
3. The phagocytic activity of normal serum–cell mixture does not differ greatly from that of immune mixtures. Only mixtures of immune serum with immune cells, however, are able to produce significant destruction of bacilli. Monocytes ingested more organisms than polymorphonuclear leukocytes. Heating the serum to 56°C for 30 min reduced bacterial killing, indicating that complement was required for optimal bactericidal activity.

More recent work has defined cellular immune functions in plague. Wong and Elberg[16] showed that immune serum contained not only antiplague antibodies but also a factor that was derived from thymus-derived lymphocytes

(T cells). This factor enhanced the resistance of mouse peritoneal macrophages to the cytotoxic effects of *Y. pestis* and enhanced the ability of these macrophages to kill bacteria. The factor appeared to be a lymphokine, and its production required both macrophages to process the immunizing antigen and T lymphocytes to produce it. In other studies of cell-mediated immunity, Wake *et al.*[17] immunized mice with *Yersinia pseudotuberculosis* and showed that long-term immunity against plague infection was correlated with a test of delayed hypersensitivity to plague vaccine.

7.1.7. Can Plague Be Eradicated?

The eradication of infectious diseases has become a desirable goal. The successful program of the WHO to eradicate smallpox in 1976 has given promise that other infections can also be eradicated. Definite progress has been made toward the eradication of measles in the United States.

The definition of eradication of an infectious disease is the interruption of transmission of that infection. Eradication cannot be used literally to mean the irretrievable death or destruction of the last infectious unit, because bacteria or viruses may lie dormant somewhere and reappear at a later time. Interruption of transmission ensures that no human or animal will contract the infection anew and, thus, the infectious disease is for practical purposes eradicated. Except for diseases like smallpox and measles, the battles against contagious diseases are usually considered to represent the more limited ambition of "control" rather than "eradiction." Nevertheless, it is useful to consider whether the possibility of eradicating plague infection is at all feasible.

Plague can be contrasted with smallpox, in order to think about the nature of an eradication effort. The features of smallpox that made its eradication a practical possibility were presented by Fenner[18] and are listed in Table 7.4. Of these eight features of smallpox, plague shares certain aspects of six, suggesting that plague could also be a target for eradication. However, the final feature of animal reservoirs is the critical difference between these diseases. The campaign against smallpox focused only on humans because there were no animal reservoirs. Thus, interrupting transmission from man to man meant that the disease was eradicated. For plague, the primary transmission to man is from rodent reservoirs, and any effort to control the disease must focus on the animal reservoirs.

TABLE 7.4
Features of Smallpox That Made This Disease a Target for Eradication and the Contrasting Features of Plague

Smallpox	Plague
Produces severe disfiguring disease that is easily identifiable	Produces fatal disease, if not treated early; typical disease is easily identifiable
Subclinical disease does not occur	Subclinical disease does occur
Not contagious in incubation period or early in disease	Usually not contagious from man to man
No problem of asymptomatic carriers	No problem of asymptomatic human carriers
Only one serotype of virus causes disease and vaccine gives immunity against the serotype	Multiple serotypes are not known to exist
Vaccine is stable to heat, not requiring cold chain for delivery to field	Killed vaccine is stable
Disease occurrence is seasonal	Disease occurrence is seasonal
No animal reservoirs of human virus are known	Disease is zoonotic in rodents and other mammals

Even if plague were not a zoonotic disease, other differences between smallpox and plague would hamper an effort at eradication. The smallpox vaccine, like other viral vaccines, is highly protective after a single dose and is nontoxic when compared to most bacterial vaccines. The killed plague vaccine, although relatively heat stable, would probably not be effective enough to confer the dramatic protection that is required in an eradiction effort.

For these reasons, plague is not considered a disease for eradication, but it needs to be controlled better. One feature of plague infection that gives control efforts a strong advantage is its geographic focality; disease activity usually remains in a restricted focus for some time, allowing workers to work intensively in the relevant places.

New research is required to find ways of interrupting transmission among rodent reservoirs. Possible approaches for the future should include the development of vaccines to be used in animals. Such vaccines would need to be nonlethal to the animals, nonpathogenic for man, transmissable among the animals by natural routes of either flea bites or by fecal–oral ingestion, and protective against the multiplication of *Y. pestis* in tissues. An alternative approach to controlling infection in rodents is the use of antibiotics. As *Y. pestis* is highly susceptible to antimicrobial drugs, rodents in certain places might be approachable by placing drugs into their food supplies and into their burrows. Although this kind of application of antimicrobial drugs to rodents' habitats would be challenging, the approach would be analogous to present efforts to apply insecticides and rodenticides in relevant places. The emergence of antimicrobial resistance in *Y. pestis* as a result of drug use would be a potential hazard of this approach.

7.2. CONTROL OF OTHER *YERSINIA* INFECTIONS

The other *Yersinia* infections, like plague, are also zoonotic infections, but the rationale of control measures is very different. Because *Yersinia enterocolitica* and *Yersinia pseudotuberculosis* are transmitted to man by the ingestion of contaminated food or water, the proper control must involve inspection of food and water sources. Investigation of outbreaks using the case–control method can often implicate the food or water source of the infection.

The most important animal reservoir for human pathogenic strains of *Y. enterocolitica* appears to be the pig. Furthermore, a survey of porcine tongue cultures by Doyle *et al.*[19] suggested that the oral cavity of pigs may be the natural reservoir of this infection. Thus, uncooked pork tongue can result in outbreaks of this disease, and the inspection of meat and periodic culturing of meat samples may be necessary for the control of this infection. Countries where pork is not consumed, as in Moslem countries of Africa and Asia, may be free of *Yersinia* infections for this reason.[20]

Two of the four outbreaks of *Y. enterocolitica* in the U.S. have been traced to the ingestion of milk.[21] These outbreaks implied that the milk was contaminated, and it is known that *Y. enterocolitica* has been cultured from raw milk. However, in both cases the culturing of milk at the dairies failed to reveal contaminated milk or a failure of pasteurization to kill *Y. enterocolitica*. Thus, it is possible that a human carrier working at the dairy contaminated the milk in these outbreaks. Studies by Francis *et al.*[22] showed that 36 strains of *Y. enterocolitica* originally cultured from raw milk in Canada were all killed at the pasteurization temperature of 62.8°C for 30 min. On the other hand, Hughes reported a heat-resistant strain of *Y. enterocolitica* in Australia,[23] and the potential problem of inadequate pasteurization should be considered during outbreaks of this disease associated with milk.

Vaccines against the rare *Yersinia* infections other than plague have not yet been developed. Nevertheless, there is considerable evidence that acquired immunity develops after infection and that this immunity can give cross-protection against other gram-negative bacterial infections. For example, Corbel[(24)] showed that formalin-killed suspensions of *Y. enterocolitica* serotype O:9 were active in evoking protective immunity in mice against challenge with virulent *Salmonella*. Thus, adults who have been exposed to variety of gram-negative bacterial infections may have crossprotective immunity against *Yersinia* infections, thus explaining the predilection of these infections for children.

REFERENCES

1. World Health Organization Informal Consultation on plague surveillance and control (Geneva, June, 1979) plague surveillance and control, *W.H.O. Chronicle* **34:**139–143 (1980).
2. P. W. Willeberg, R. Ruppanner, D. E. Behymer, H. H. Higa, C. E. Franti, R. A. Thompson, and B. Bohannan, Epidemiologic survey of sylvatic plague by serotesting coyote sentinels with enzyme immunoassay, *Am. J. Epidemiol.* **110:**328–334 (1979).
3. D. C. Cavanaugh, B. D. Thorpe, J. B. Bushman, P. S. Nicholes, and J. H. Rust, Detection of an enzootic plague focus by serological methods, *Bull. W.H.O.* **32:**197–203 (1965).
4. J. E. Brooks, P. T. Htun, and H. Naing, The susceptibility of *Bandicota bengalensis* from Rangoon, Burma, to several anticoagulant rodenticides, *J. Hyg.* **84:**127–135 (1980).
5. J. E. Brooks and P. T. Htun, Laboratory evaluation of scilliroside used as a rodenticide against the lesser bandicoot rat, *Bandicota bengalensis, J. Hyg.* **85:**227–234, (1980).

5a. J. M. Mann, W. J. Martone, J. M. Boyce, A. F. Kaufman, A. M. Barnes, and N. S. Weber, Endemic human plague in New Mexico: Risk factors associated with acquisition of infection, *J. Infect. Dis.* **140:**397–401 (1979).

6. K. F. Meyer, Effectiveness of live or killed plague vaccines in man. *Bull. W.H.O.* **42:**653–666 (1970).
7. K. F. Meyer, D. C. Cavanaugh, P. J. Bartelloni, and J. D. Marshall. Plage immunization I. Past and present trends, *J. Infect. Dis.* **129**(Suppl.):513–518 (1974).
8. D. C. Cavanaugh, B. L. Elisberg, C. H. Llewellyn, J. D. Marshall, J. H. Rust, J. E. Williams, and K. F. Meyer, Plague immunization V. Indirect evidence for the efficacy of plague vaccine, *J. Infect. Dis.* **129**(Suppl):537–540 (1974).
9. N. V. Liem and M. Jullien, Present status of plague vaccine and its problems, Symposium on Plague, Saigon, Vietnam (1970).
10. T. Butler and B. W. Hudson, The serological response to *Yersinia pestis* infection, *Bull. W.H.O.* **55:**39–42 (1977).
11. Plague vaccine, *Morbidity and Morality, Weekly Report* **31:**301–304 (1982).
12. J. E. Williams and D. C. Cavanaugh, Measuring the efficacy of vaccination in affording protection against plague, *Bull. W.H.O.* **57**(2):309–313 (1979).
13. T. H. Chen, S. S. Elberg, and D. M. Eisler, Immunity in plague: Protection of the vervet *(Cercopithecus aethiops)* against pneumonic plague by oral administration of live attenuated *Yersinia pestis, J. Infect. Dis.* **135:**289–293 (1977).

14. J. M. Alonso, B. Hurtrel, D. Mazigh, M. A. Chalvignac, and H. H. Mollaret, Temperature-modulated immunogenicity to *Yersinia pestis* from *Yersinia enterocolitica 03*, *Infect. Immun.* **36:**423–425 (1982).
15. E. Jawetz and K. F. Meyer, Studies on plague immunity in experimental animals II. Some factors of the immunity mechanism in bubonic plague, *J. Immunol.* **49:**15–30 (1944).
16. J. F. Wong and S. S. Elberg, Cellular immune response to *Yersinia pestis* modulated by products from thymus-derived lymphocytes, *J. Infect. Dis.* **135:**67–78 (1977).
17. A. Wake, H. Morita, and M. Wake, Mechanisms of long- and short-term immunity to plague, *Immunology* **34:**1045–1052 (1978).
18. F. Fenner, Global eradication of smallpox. *Rev. Infect. Dis.* **4:**916–922 (1982).
19. M. P. Doyle, M. B. Hugdahl, and S. L. Taylor, Isolation of virulent *Yersinia enterocolitica* from porcine tongues, *Appl. Environ. Microbiol.* **42:**661–666 (1981).
20. A. R. Samadi, K. Wachsmuth, M. I. Huq, M. Mahbub, and D. E. Agbonlahor, An attempt to detect *Yersinia enterocolitica* in Dacca, Bangladesh, *Trop. Geogr. Med.* **34:**151–154 (1982).
21. Multi-state outbreak of yersiniosis, *Morbidity and Mortality Weekly Report* **31:**505–506 (1982).
22. D. W. Francis, P. L. Spaulding, J. Lovett, Enterotoxin production and thermal resistance of *Yersinia enterocolitica* in milk, *Appl. Environ. Microbiol.* **40:**174–176 (1980).
23. D. Hughes, Isolation of *Yersinia enterocolitica* from milk and a dairy in Australia, *J. Appl. Bacteriol.* **46:**125–130 (1979).
24. M. J. Corbel, Stimulation of protective immunity to *Salmonella* Kauffmann-White group N serotypes by *Brucella abortus* and *Yersinia enterocolitica* antigens, *Br. Vet. J.* **131:**625–626 (1975).

Index